Intestinal Microbiome: Functional Aspects in Health and Disease

Nestlé Nutrition Institute Workshop Series

Vol. 88

Intestinal Microbiome: Functional Aspects in Health and Disease

Editors

Erika Isolauri Turku

Philip M. Sherman Toronto, ON

W. Allan Walker Charlestown, MA

KARGER

Nestlé Nutrition Institute

Nestec Ltd., 55 Avenue Nestlé, CH–1800 Vevey (Switzerland)
S. Karger AG, P.O. Box, CH–4009 Basel (Switzerland) www.karger.com

Library of Congress Cataloging-in-Publication Data

Names: Nestlé Nutrition Workshop (88th : 2016 : Playa del Carmen, Mexico), author. | Isolauri, Erika, editor. | Sherman, Philip M., editor. | Walker, W. Allan, editor.
Title: Intestinal microbiome : functional aspects in health and disease / editors, Erika Isolauri, Philip M. Sherman, W. Allan Walker.
Description: Basel ; New York : Karger, [2017] | Series: Nestlé Nutrition Institute workshop series, ISSN 1664-2147 ; vol. 88 | Includes bibliographical references and index.
Identifiers: LCCN 2017010377| ISBN 9783318060300 (hard cover : alk. paper) | ISBN 9783318060317 (electronic version)
Subjects: | MESH: Gastrointestinal Microbiome--physiology | Fetal Development | Infant | Intestines--microbiology | Congresses
Classification: LCC RC816 | NLM WI 102 | DDC 616.3/3--dc23 LC record available at https://lccn.loc.gov/2017010377

Printed on acid-free and non-aging paper (ISO 9706)
ISBN 978–3–318–06030–0
e-ISBN 978–3–318–06031–7
ISSN 1664–2147
e-ISSN 1664–2155

KARGER Basel · Freiburg · Paris · London · New York · Chennai · New Delhi · Bangkok · Beijing · Shanghai · Tokyo · Kuala Lumpur · Singapore · Sydney

Contents

For more information on related publications, please consult the NNI website: www.nestlenutrition-institute.org

Preface

Over the last decade, major attention in clinical research has been focused on the importance of the intestinal microbiome in health and disease. This is of particular importance during the first thousand days of life (from conception until 2 years of age) when the newborn infant has to adjust to the extrauterine environment. It is now apparent that exposure to microbes in utero represents an important initial impact on fetal development, in part through epigenetic processes. The nature of the pregnant mother's health impacts on the fetus through microbiota in the maternal gut entering the blood stream and traversing through the placenta to access the amniotic fluid.

The mother's intestinal microbiome changes during pregnancy, particularly during the third trimester, principally under hormonal influences. This also has an impact on fetal microbial exposure. The nature of delivery (cesarean section vs. vaginal delivery) and perinatal antibiotic treatment can influence initial microbial colonization and the development of appropriate intestinal defense mechanisms which, in turn, can affect the expression of disease (e.g., allergy, autoimmune disease, and brain function) later in life. Current research is underway to determine whether the microbiota or metabolic changes are primary, causative factors in the complex interrelationships.

As mentioned, modification of the intrauterine environment can affect fetal development. We now know that microbes and their metabolites can influence fetal development by epigenetic mechanisms. The nature of initial colonization influences newborn infants at a time when the newborn is developing defenses. Appropriate colonization is associated with healthy immune defense mechanisms, whereas inappropriate colonization (dysbiosis) can result in immune-mediated disease in later life. Diseases associated with dysbiosis at birth include necrotizing enterocolitis, obesity, allergy, functional bowel disorders, and impaired mental health.

An important environmental factor influencing the nature of colonization is diet. At no time in life is diet more important than during the colonization that is part of the postpartum period. Exclusive breast feeding for 4–6 months in conjunction with full-term vaginal delivery without antibiotics is the ideal setting for normal initial bacterial colonization and appropriate development of host defenses. Oligosaccharides contained in human breast milk (nondigestible complex carbohydrates) have a profound effect on intestinal microbiota and their metabolites. These major constituents of breast milk provide nutrition for the stimulation of health by promoting bacteria and release of short-chain fatty acids as well as other metabolites which can influence immune function towards immune homeostasis, including the development of tolerance to innocuous antigens and commensal bacteria. These complex carbohydrates can also interact with pathogenic bacteria and viruses within the intestine to prevent disease and have a direct impact on enterocyte and lymphocyte responses to microbial invasion. In this Nestlé Workshop, the importance of microbiota in the setting of both health and disease has been addressed.

Erika Isolauri
Philip M. Sherman
W. Allan Walker

Foreword

The importance and role of gut microbiota in human health and disease are topics attracting research interest and attention in clinical practice during the last decades. A large number of bacteria and microbes invade the infant's gut during the first days and weeks of their life. Neonatal gut microbiota establishment represents a crucial stage in gut maturation and metabolic and immunologic programming, and, consequently, affects the short- and long-term health status.

The 88th Nestlé Nutrition Institute Workshop entitled "Intestinal Microbiome: Functional Aspects in Health and Disease" was held in Playa del Carmen (Mexico) on September 22–25, 2016.

We have chosen an incredible international faculty led by distinguished Chairmen: *Prof. W. Allan Walker* (Conrad Taff Professor of Nutrition and Pediatrics, Harvard Medical School, USA); *Prof. Erika Isolauri* (Head of the Department of Clinical Medicine, University of Turku, Finland); and *Prof. Philip M. Sherman* (Hospital for Sick Children, University of Toronto, Canada).

The first session on the Evolution of human microbiota, chaired by *Prof. W. Allan Walker*, was focused on the development of the human microbiome and the importance of normal colonization of the newborn gut in immune development and disease prevention. The speakers have presented available scientific data supporting a role of microbial changes during pregnancy and infancy for a healthy start in life. Special focus was given to existing evidence of environmental factors (e.g. diet, nutrition, and infections) on human health and epigenetic mechanisms which could provide a plausible framework for the development of many multifactorial diseases, including inflammatory bowel disease. The session has also illuminated a crucial role of the gut microbiota in bidirectional brain-gut interactions and the potential role of the brain-gut axis in influencing health and behavior.

The second session with *Prof. Erika Isolauri* demonstrated a link between basic research and science and its clinical implications. The experts highlighted the clinical practice and environmental interference in the development of normal gut microbiota as well as clinical conditions associated with dysbiosis. The speakers presented scientific evidence on dysbiosis in the neonatal period, particularly on the role of preterm birth and cesarean section deliveries, the role of microbiota in the development of necrotizing enterocolitis, and a correlation between environmental factors/antibiotic exposure during critical periods of early infancy and the development of obesity in later life. The importance of microbiota in functional gastrointestinal disorders and the role of diet and microbiota in health and disease was also highlighted during the session.

The third session with *Prof. Philip M. Sherman* covered various aspects of human milk evolution and human milk oligosaccharides (HMOs). The presentations on basic science and compositional analysis of identified HMOs help us to understand their mechanisms in modulating the gut microbiome, potential effects on immune functions, and their future role in infant nutrition. Current scientific evidence and clinical research findings support the importance of HMOs in early nutrition and pave the way for future opportunities and regulatory framework to include HMOs in infant formula.

We appreciate all participants who have contributed to formal and informal discussions during the workshop.

We would like to acknowledge all those who have been involved in the workshop organization either at global or regional level; we especially thank Dr. Salvador Villalpando and his team for the wonderful workshop organization.

Dr. Natalia Wagemans
Head of the Nestlé Nutrition Institute
Vevey, Switzerland

Contributors

Chairpersons & Speakers

Assist. Prof. Meghan Azad
Department of Pediatrics and Child Health
Children's Hospital Research Institute of Manitoba
501G John Buhler Research Center
715 McDermot Avenue
Winnipeg, MB R3E 3P4
Canada
E-Mail meghan.azad@umanitoba.ca

Prof. J. Bruce German
Foods for Health Institute
University of California, Davis
1 Shields Avenue
Davis CA 95616
USA
E-Mail jbgerman@ucdavis.edu

Prof. Erika Isolauri
Department of Clinical Medicine
University of Turku
Kiinamyllynkatu 10
C-Wing, 7th Floor
FI–20520 Turku
Finland
E-Mail eriiso@utu.fi

Dr. Omry Koren
Faculty of Medicine
Bar-Ilan University
8 Henrietta Szold Street
Safed 1311502
Israel
E-Mail Omry.Koren@biu.ac.il

Prof. Dr. Clemens Kunz
Institute of Nutritional Sciences
Justus Liebig University Giessen
Wilhelmstreet 20
DE–35392 Giessen
Germany
E-Mail clemens.kunz@uni-giessen.de

Dr. Emeran A. Mayer
G. Oppenheimer Center for Neurobiology of Stress and Resilience
Vatche and Tamar Manoukian Division of Digestive Diseases
David Geffen School of Medicine at UCLA
CHS 42-210 MC737818
10833 Le Conte Avenue
Los Angeles, CA 90095-7378
USA
E-Mail emayer@ucla.edu

Prof. David A. Mills
Department of Food Science and Technology
University of California
1 Shields Avenue
3142 RMI North Building
Davis, CA 95616-5270
USA
E-Mail damills@ucdavis.edu

Prof. Josef Neu
Division of Neonatology
Department of Pediatrics
University of Florida
1600 SW Archer Road
Human Development Building
Room HD 112
Gainesville, FL 32610
USA
E-Mail neuj@peds.ufl.edu

Prof. Sanjay Patole
Department of Neonatal Paediatrics
KEM Hospital for Women
374 Bagot Road, Subiaco
Perth, WA 6008
Australia
E-Mail sanjay.patole@health.wa.gov.au

Dr. Samuli Rautava
Department of Pediatrics
Turku University Hospital
University of Turku
Kiinamyllynkatu 4–8
FI–20520 Turku
Finland
E-Mail samulirautava@gmail.com

Prof. Seppo Salminen
Functional Foods Forum
Faculty of Medicine
University of Turku
FI–20014 Turku
Finland
E-Mail seppo.salminen@utu.fi

Dr. Ting-Chin David Shen
Division of Gastroenterology
Perelman School of Medicine
University of Pennsylvania
914 Biomedical Research Building II/III
421 Curie Boulevard
Philadelphia, PA 19104
USA
E-Mail david.shen@uphs.upenn.edu

Prof. Philip M. Sherman
Hospital for Sick Children
University of Toronto
555 University Avenue
Toronto, ON M5G 1X8
Canada
E-Mail philip.sherman@sickkids.ca

Prof. W. Allan Walker
Mucosal Immunology and Biology
Research Center
MassGeneral Hospital for Children
114 16th Street (114-3503)
Charlestown, MA 02129-4404
USA
E-Mail wwalker@partners.org

Dr. Matthias Zilbauer
Department of Paediatrics
University of Cambridge
Level 8 Addenbrooke's Hospital
Box 116
Hills Road
Cambridge CB2 0QQ
UK
E-Mail mz304@medschl.cam.ac.uk

Participants

Frances Connor /Australia
Avi Lemberg/Australia
Ferdinand Haschke/Austria
Farid Ahmed/Bangladesh
Syed Khairul Amin/Bangladesh
Claudia Gasparian/Brazil
Fernanda Rodrigues/Brazil
Macarena Derado Becker/Chile
Martin Marie Bruno Gotteland/Chile
Wilson Daza/Colombia
Carolina Castellanos/Dominican Republic
Yajaira Cruz/Dominican Republic
Frank Inoa/Dominican Republic
Jenny Kranwinkel/Dominican Republic
Yanet Nuñez/Dominican Republic
Angela Sanchez/Dominican Republic
Cecilia Cedeño/Ecuador
Fernando Montaño/Ecuador
Alfredo Naranjo/Ecuador
Axel Enninger/Germany
Mike Possner/Germany
Jorge Palacios/Guatemala
Khaled Alsaeid/Kuwait
Naji Doumit/Lebanon
Bassam Eid/Lebanon
Carlos Patricio Acosta Rodriguez Bueno/Mexico
Rocio Gabriela Aguiñaga Villaseñor/Mexico
Aristoteles Alvarez Gonzalez/Mexico
Rafael Alvarez Gonzalez/Mexico

Liliana Arroyo Cruz/Mexico
Ana Basaguren/Mexico
Diego Battaglia Velazquez/Mexico
Daniella Bautista/Mexico
Daniela Bervera/Mexico
Lourdes Cahuich/Mexico
Elia Noemi Camacho Ojeda/Mexico
Arturo Cardona Pérez/Mexico
Juana Elvia Castillo Calderón/Mexico
Adrian Ceballos Bocanegra/Mexico
José Antonio Chavez Barrera/Mexico
Yazmin Chirinó Barceló/Mexico
Dino Roberto Pietropaolo Cienfuegos/Mexico
Alejandra Coronado Sarco/Mexico
Joshue Covarrubias Esquer/Mexico
Claudia de la Vega/Mexico
Dagoberto Delgado Franco/Mexico
Yael Encinas Bravo/Mexico
Salvador Espino Y Sosa/Mexico
Isaac Estrada/Mexico
Guadalupe del Carmen Estrada Gutierrez/Mexico
Judith Flores Calderón
Luis Octavio Flores Romo/Mexico
Raúl Garza Bulnes/Mexico
Rocco José González Morán/Mexico
Mariana Herrera Pen/Mexico
Patricia Laureant Ibarra/Mexico
Maria de Luz Irache/Mexico
Maria de Luz Iracheta Jerez/Mexico
Ulises Leal Quiroga/Mexico
Lourdes Lemus Varela/Mexico
Veronica López Guevara/Mexico
Javier López Morales/Mexico
Monica Martina Luna/Mexico
Jose de Jesús Magaña Mungia/Mexico
Luis Alberto Mendez Trujeque/Mexico
Luciano Mendiola/Mexico
Luis Gustavo Orozco Alatorre/Mexico
Alberto Orozco Gutierrez/Mexico
Diana Paulina Orozco Romero/Mexico
Penelope Ortal Vite/Mexico
Arturo Perea Martinez/Mexico
Adriana Pinzon Navarro/Mexico
Rafael Ponce de León Barajas/Mexico
Luz Angelica Ramiréz García/Mexico
Jose Nicolas Reynes Manzur/Mexico
Carlos Gilberto Alonso Rivera/Mexico
Alicia Robledo Galvan/Mexico
Efren Rodriguez/Mexico
Ameyalli Rodriguez Cano/Mexico
Silvia Romero Maldonado/Mexico
Marlene Ruiz Castillo/Mexico
Abel Salazar Martínez/Mexico
Roberto Flores Santos/Mexico
Alejandro Serrano Sierra/Mexico
Claudia Sifuentes Vela/Mexico

Neri Solis Perales/Mexico
Mariana Tirado/Mexico
Martín Vargas Acevedo/Mexico
Francisco Vargas Quintal/Mexico
Edgar Vazquez Garibay/Mexico
Pilar Vazquez/Mexico
Salvador Villalpando Carrión/Mexico
Juan José Carpio Cornejo/Perú
José Gonzáles Benavides/Perú
Ángel Muñoz Ortega/Perú
Pierina Queirolo Rivera/Perú
Yuri Valencia Yabar/Perú
Luis Alberto Yalta Ramírez/Perú
Victoria Hurduc/Romania
Sorin-Claudiu Man/Romania
Laura Trandafir/Romania
Grace Uy/Singapore
Mª Carmen Collado/Spain
Marisa Vidal/Spain
Robert Di Gregorio/Switzerland
Sanjeev Ganguly/Switzerland
Karina Negro/Switzerland
Jose Saavedra/Switzerland
Evelyn Spivey-Krobath/Switzerland
Marco Turini/Switzerland
Lateefa Rashedalmarzooqi/United Arab Emirates
Mohamed Salah/United Arab Emirates
Jodi Bettler/USA
Jayne Davies/USA
Melissa Marko/USA
Kathryn Pramuk/USA
María José Castro/Venezuela
María Eugenia Reymundez/Venezuela
Rafael Santiago/Venezuela

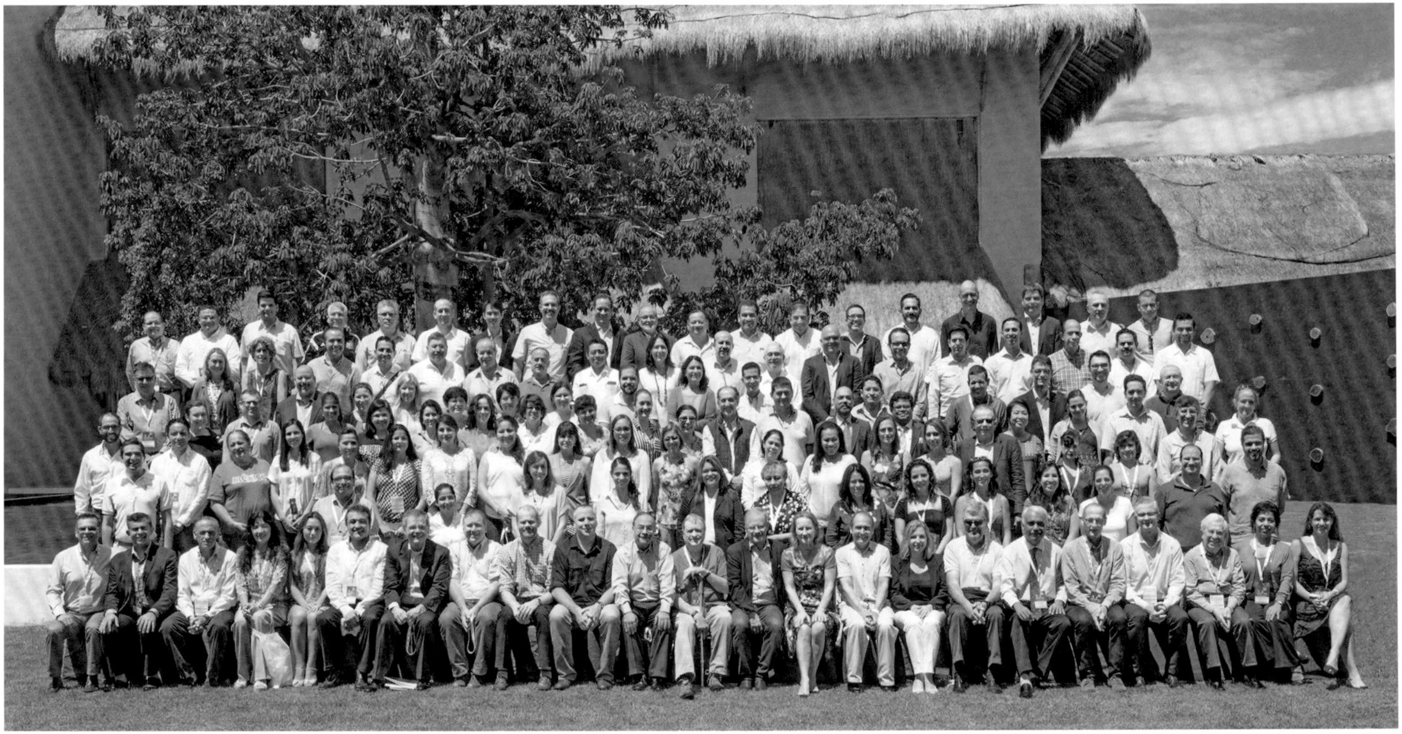

88th Nestlé Nutrition Institute Workshop
Playa del Carmen, Mexico, September 22–25, 2016

Isolauri E, Sherman PM, Walker WA (eds): Intestinal Microbiome: Functional Aspects in Health and Disease. Nestlé Nutr Inst Workshop Ser, vol 88, pp 1–9, (DOI: 10.1159/000455207)

The Pregnancy Microbiome

Hadar Neuman • Omry Koren

Faculty of Medicine, Bar-Ilan University, Safed, Israel

Abstract

In recent years, microbiome research has revealed multiple essential roles of the microorganisms residing within the human body in host metabolism, immunity, and overall health. Numerous physiological and pathological states, including obesity and the metabolic syndrome, have been correlated with microbial changes, termed dysbiosis. Our microbiomes change in response to our environment, diet, weight, hormones, and other factors. It is, therefore, not surprising that there are also significant changes in the microbiome during pregnancy when dramatic weight gain and metabolic and immunological changes occur. In this review, we summarize the known changes in microbial composition throughout pregnancy at a variety of body sites, including the gut, vagina, oral cavity, and placenta, and we describe several studies that have linked pregnancy complications with microbial changes. Unlike the case of certain disease states, such as obesity, where dysbiosis is considered to have negative effects, we believe that the microbial alterations observed during pregnancy are vital for a healthy pregnancy. While more research in this field is required to reveal specific mechanisms and pathways regulating these alterations, the microbial changes during pregnancy are likely coordinated with the immune, endocrine, and metabolic states.

Introduction

The human microbiome includes hundreds of different microbial species residing within and on us, playing essential roles in our metabolism and immune and endocrine system. These microbial populations have been shown to change during our lifetime, from infancy to childhood, adulthood, and old age.

The microbial populations are also highly affected by weight gain, diet, and immune and hormonal changes. Therefore, it is not surprising that there are distinct alterations in the microbiota at multiple sites within the body during pregnancy. Pregnancy, a complex physiological process, is associated with simultaneous hormonal changes, weight gain, and immune system modulations, which must all be synchronized to preserve the health of both the mother and the offspring [1]. In this review, we describe the pronounced microbial changes that occur in the pregnant female. We hypothesize that an appropriate microbiota is essential for the healthy early development of the fetus and pregnancy maintenance. Moreover, we suggest that the microbial changes during pregnancy are highly correlated with other physiological changes, including those in hormones, immunity, and metabolism. Understanding the roles of the microbiome throughout pregnancy in health and disease is of great importance for opening new research avenues and suggesting new therapeutic approaches. Yet, there remains much to be discovered regarding the precise microbial alterations during pregnancy, their timing, and, potentially, their further effects.

Studying the microbiota in pregnancy opens another fascinating question of whether the fetus is exposed to microbes, and, if so, at what stage of development. While it has been thought for over a century that we are born germ free [2], numerous pieces of evidence now cast doubt on this hypothesis and suggest that a bacterial presence already exists in the fetoplacental unit [3, 4]. The enigma of whether a placental microbiota exists as well is still not fully resolved.

The Healthy Microbiome

The human microbiome is a collection of bacteria, archaea, fungi, and viruses, all residing within our bodies and including their genetic material. Within each one of us, there are trillions of microbial cells representing hundreds of different species. Together, they play important roles in host metabolism, immunity, endocrinology [5], and overall health. The microbial compositions vary between people and are greatly affected by diet, additional environmental factors, weight gain, and immune state, etc. Different body sites harbor different microbial populations due to varying levels of pH, oxygen, nutrients, humidity, and temperature [5]. Therefore, the gut, oral cavity, and vagina each harbor distinct bacterial communities, potentially playing different beneficial roles. In this review, we mainly discuss alterations during pregnancy in bacterial communities of the microbiome, as these are the best studied to date. It is important to remember that pregnancy is a healthy physiological process in which beneficial microbial alterations are expected. This is in contrast to disease states such as obesity, inflammatory bowel disease (IBD), diabetes, and the metabolic syndrome, in which an unhealthy shift in microbiota composition, termed dysbiosis, may occur [5].

Factors Affecting the Microbiota during Pregnancy

One group of initial changes that occur during pregnancy is hormonal changes. Most importantly, progesterone and estrogen levels rise dramatically, with numerous physiological effects. These hormonal levels are likely to affect the microbiome composition since it has previously been shown that microbial components can respond to and regulate host hormones, and that host hormones influence bacterial growth. On the other hand, the microbiota can also produce and secrete hormones, emphasizing the bidirectional nature of the interplay between microbiota and hormones. Nonetheless, direct effects of progesterone and estrogen on the microbiota, and the effects of the microbiota on these hormones, have not yet been proven [6].

Additionally, significant immune changes occur during pregnancy, and these are likely to affect the microbiota. The immune changes are complex in order to protect the fetus and mother from infection on the one hand, while nevertheless enabling fetal immune development and preventing fetal rejection by the maternal immune system. The microbial components are crucial players in this immune modulation; however, they themselves are also affected by immune changes.

Finally, metabolic changes occur during pregnancy, including changes in energy homeostasis, fat storage, and hormonal regulation. In many ways, the metabolic changes associated with pregnancy are similar to those that occur in the metabolic syndrome, including weight gain, elevated fasting blood glucose levels, insulin resistance, glucose intolerance, low-grade inflammation, and changes in metabolic hormone levels [7]. While the microbiota plays active roles in these metabolic processes, it is also highly affected by host metabolism, as seen by dysbiosis in obesity, the metabolic syndrome, and diabetes. Therefore, the metabolic changes occurring during pregnancy are expected to influence the microbiota composition.

Pregnancy Leads to Changes in the Gut Microbiota

Several alterations in the gut microbiota have been associated with pregnancy progression. In general, pregnancy is characterized by an increase in the bacterial load and profound alterations in the composition of the gut microbiota [7]. Most of the changes relative to nonpregnant women are seen in late pregnancy. These dramatic changes are characterized by reduced individual richness (α diversity), increased between-subject diversity (β diversity), and alterations in abundance of certain species [8]. Increased abundance of members of the Actinobacteria and Proteobacteria phyla are observed at the expense of reduced abundance of *Faecalibacterium* and other short-chain fatty-acid producers. *Faecalibacterium* is a butyrate-producing bacterium with anti-inflammatory activities, which is depleted in metabolic syndrome patients [9]. This is of particular interest, since pregnancy shares some characteristics with the metabolic syndrome, including weight gain, insulin insensitivity, and higher levels of low-grade inflammatory markers [8]. However, in contrast to metabolic syndrome patients, in the context of pregnancy, these parameters are normal requirements for healthy fetal development. Further comparisons between the microbial signatures of pregnancy and disease states such as the metabolic syndrome may highlight common as well as unique pathways and microbial involvement in each condition.

When starting to dissect the roles of the gut microbiota during pregnancy, the third-trimester microbiota was shown to cause increased weight gain, insulin resistance, and a greater inflammatory response compared to the first-trimester microbiota when transferred to germ-free mice [8]. These findings demonstrate that the microbial components actively contribute to changes in host immunology as well as metabolism. Gut microbiota have also been suggested to play a role in host weight gain during pregnancy via increased absorption of glucose and fatty acids, increased fasting-induced adipocyte factor secretion, induction of catabolic pathways, and stimulation of the immune system [8, 10].

Since the microbial communities are greatly affected by the host diet and initial weight, the microbiota of pregnant women differ accordingly [10]. Overweight pregnant women exhibit significantly higher levels of gut *Bacteroides* and *Staphylococcus* than pregnant women of normal weight [10]. While most studies show significant alterations in gut microbiota during pregnancy, DiGiulio et al. [11] did not detect any changes in gut or vaginal microbiota composition including richness indexes during gestation.

Antibiotics administered during pregnancy were shown to affect the microbiome composition and diversity, as well as to promote weight gain in rodents [12]. It is especially intriguing to understand the consequences of the maternal microbiome composition during pregnancy on the offspring in terms of weight gain, immunity, and infant health [13]. Recently, the maternal microbiota was shown to shape the offspring's immune system in terms of immune gene expression and numbers of innate cells [14], and it was also hypothesized that microbial exposure during pregnancy may be of great importance for preventing allergic disease in the offspring [15].

Pregnancy Leads to Changes in the Vaginal Microbiota

The vaginal microbiome undergoes significant changes during pregnancy as well [7], including a significant decrease in overall diversity, increased stability, and increased abundance of *Lactobacillus* species [16]. *Lactobacillus* species are lactic acid-producing bacteria that normally dominate the vaginal microbiota. Their increase during pregnancy correlates with a decrease in the vaginal pH, creating a barrier against pathogenic bacteria and viral infections, and an increase in vaginal secretions [17, 18]. The major changes in the vaginal microbial compositions occur in early pregnancy, while the communities at the later stages of pregnancy resemble those of the nonpregnant state [16]. In pregnancy, there is often a dominant *Lactobacillus* species, although the specific species varies according to the ethnic group [19, 20]. As expected, during the postpartum period, the vaginal microbiome gradually reverts to baseline characteristics, including a decrease in *Lactobacillus* species abundance, an increase in α diversity, and enrichment of bacteria associated with vaginosis, such as Actinobacteria [19].

Pregnancy Leads to Changes in the Oral Microbiota

The main change occurring in the oral microbiota during pregnancy is an increase in the microbial load. A study which compared the abundance of 7 common bacterial species in the oral cavity of nonpregnant women and women at different stages of pregnancy found that the total viable microbial counts were higher during pregnancy, as were levels of the pathogenic bacteria *Porphyromonas gingivalis* and *Aggregatibacter actinomycetemcomitans,* and *Candida* [21].

It remains to be discovered how pregnancy leads to changes in the oral composition. There have also been several studies that found correlations between oral infections and pregnancy complications, further suggesting mechanisms connecting the oral microbiome with the state of pregnancy. One explanation for the increased oral microbial load may be the overall immune changes (suppression) during pregnancy.

Debate over the Placental Microbiota

Until recently, the fetoplacental unit was considered to be germ free, and the first exposure to microbes was assumed to occur during delivery. Accordingly, any signs of bacteria in the placenta or embryonic fluids were considered to be a result of contamination originating from the lower genital tract and posing a potential danger to the pregnancy [22]. However, with the recent leap in understanding the complexity of our microbiota and its important roles in healthy states, multiple studies have tried to examine whether a healthy placental microbiota exists. Several findings using both culture and metagenomic techniques suggest the presence of bacteria in the healthy placenta. First, bacteria have been cultured from placentas of healthy women without chorioamnionitis [23]. Furthermore, using whole-genome shotgun sequencing of samples from 320 subjects, Aagaard et al. [4] reported that the placenta contains a unique microbiome, somewhat resembling the oral one. This similarity between the oral and placental microbiota may be less surprising than it initially appears, since periodontal infections have previously been linked to an increased risk of pregnancy complications [7]. One hypothesis is that bacteria may pass from the oral cavity to the placenta through an unknown mechanism. In contrast, other studies highly doubt the presence of a placental microbiome, since even when such colonization is found, it is of extremely low biomass and may therefore represent contamination rather than a real phenomenon. It was in fact shown that low-biomass samples many times resemble contamination controls due to commercial reagents, as opposed to unique placental microbiota [24]. Such technical contaminations are especially prevalent when placental samples are received following natural births, when contaminations from the birth canal are likely.

As for amniotic fluid, a number of studies have shown the presence of microbes in healthy women using cultivation and PCR techniques [13]. Additionally, it was claimed that the bacterial populations detected in meconium might represent prenatal bacterial exposure. This may explain differences in microbial compositions found in meconium between infants of mothers who received probiotics during pregnancy compared to controls [25].

The debate over the placental microbiome remains an intriguing, open question. If indeed future research will verify the existence of these populations, further studies should investigate the potential roles of microbiota in gestation and fetal development.

Pregnancy Complications Are Correlated with Dysbiosis and Infections

Pregnancy complications occur commonly (usually with unknown etiology), are observed in approximately 1 in every 6 pregnancies, and pose a serious risk for both maternal and fetal health and survival [26]. The most common pregnancy complications include preeclampsia, eclampsia, intrauterine growth restriction, and preterm birth. While some bacterial infections have been correlated with pregnancy complications, precise causal mechanisms are, as yet, unknown [27]. Several more recent studies have attempted to test for correlations between the microbial communities present during pregnancy and pregnancy complications [28].

Two studies demonstrated a correlation between high α (within-individual) diversity in gut microbiota and preterm birth [20], while a third study did not [29]. Additionally, certain vaginal communities in early pregnancy stages were significantly associated with an elevated rate of preterm birth [11]. These communities include higher abundances of *Gardnerella* and *Ureaplasma*, lower abundances of *Lactobacillus* sp., and higher α diversity. Additionally, the presence of certain vaginal fungi, even when asymptomatic, such as *Candida albicans*, is correlated with higher rates of preterm birth [30].

Finally, oral infections have been reported as risk factors for pregnancy complications such as preterm birth [31, 32]. There are several theories regarding potential mechanisms for this effect, including the direct contact with microbiota via the placenta or more systemic inflammation and hormone production leading to preterm birth [4, 33, 34].

Conclusions

In this review, we discuss the dramatic changes observed in the microbiome composition at multiple sites (gut, vagina, oral cavity, and placenta) during healthy pregnancy and in complicated pregnancy. We try to present these changes in the context of the overall unique physiology during pregnancy. Pregnancy is a natural process of growth and development, in which many physiological changes occur, including changes in body composition, weight gain, hormonal levels, inflammation, and metabolic states. These multiple changes have distinct effects on the microbiota, which is altered accordingly. These changes are finely synchronized to ensure the healthy development of the embryo and fetus, and to meet the growing needs of the fetus up to delivery.

The debate over the sterile fetus has not been resolved. While some studies provide evidence for the presence of bacteria in the placenta, others contradict this, claiming that the bacteria observed were introduced by contamination. Additional studies are, therefore, required to resolve this issue. The possibility of early microbial colonization of the fetus suggests that from the very beginning of development, there may be reciprocal interactions between the developing host and microbiota, and that maternal microbial components may be transferred very early in development.

Future research will likely reveal the interactions and pathways linking the various physiological changes to the microbial changes, thereby explaining the significance of each change observed. Such studies may also have clinical relevance in terms of recommendations for antibiotic treatments, probiotics, and potential therapies for pregnancy complications.

Disclosure Statement

The authors declare that no financial or other conflict of interest exists in relation to the contents of the chapter.

References

1 Dunlop AL, Mulle JG, Ferranti EP, et al: Maternal microbiome and pregnancy outcomes that impact infant health: a review. Adv Neonatal Care 2015;15:377–385.

2 Tissier H: Recherches sur la flore intestinale des nourrissons (état normal et pathologique); thesis, University of Paris, 1900.

3 Hu J, Nomura Y, Bashir A, et al: Diversified microbiota of meconium is affected by maternal diabetes status. PLoS One 2013; 8:e78257.

4 Aagaard K, Ma J, Antony KM, et al: The placenta harbors a unique microbiome. Sci Transl Med 2014;6:237ra65.

5 Spor A, Koren O, Ley R: Unravelling the effects of the environment and host genotype on the gut microbiome. Nat Rev Microbiol 2011;9:279–290.

6 Neuman H, Debelius JW, Knight R, Koren O: Microbial endocrinology: the interplay between the microbiota and the endocrine system. FEMS Microbiol Rev 2015;39:509–521.

7 Nuriel-Ohayon M, Neuman H, Koren O: Microbial changes during pregnancy, birth, and infancy. Front Microbiol 2016;7:1031.

8 Koren O, Goodrich JK, Cullender TC, et al: Host remodeling of the gut microbiome and metabolic changes during pregnancy. Cell 2012;150:470–480.

9 Haro C, Garcia-Carpintero S, Alcala-Diaz JF, et al: The gut microbial community in metabolic syndrome patients is modified by diet. J Nutr Biochem 2016;27:27–31.

10 Collado MC, Isolauri E, Laitinen K, Salminen S: Distinct composition of gut microbiota during pregnancy in overweight and normal-weight women. Am J Clin Nutr 2008;88:894–899.

11 DiGiulio DB, Callahan BJ, McMurdie PJ, et al: Temporal and spatial variation of the human microbiota during pregnancy. Proc Natl Acad Sci U S A 2015;112:11060–11065.

12 Khan I, Azhar EI, Abbas AT, et al: Metagenomic analysis of antibiotic-induced changes in gut microbiota in a pregnant rat model. Front Pharmacol 2016;7:104.

13 Kuperman AA, Koren O: Antibiotic use during pregnancy: how bad is it? BMC Med 2016;14:91.

14 Gomez de Aguero M, Ganal-Vonarburg SC, Fuhrer T, et al: The maternal microbiota drives early postnatal innate immune development. Science 2016;351:1296–1302.

15 Abrahamsson TR, Wu RY, Jenmalm MC: Gut microbiota and allergy: the importance of the pregnancy period. Pediatr Res 2015;77: 214–219.

16 Aagaard K, Riehle K, Ma J, et al: A metagenomic approach to characterization of the vaginal microbiome signature in pregnancy. PLoS One 2012;7:e36466.

17 Ravel J, Gajer P, Abdo Z, et al: Vaginal microbiome of reproductive-age women. Proc Natl Acad Sci U S A 2011;108(suppl 1):4680–4687.

18 Prince AL, Antony KM, Ma J, Aagaard KM: The microbiome and development: a mother's perspective. Semin Reprod Med 2014;32: 14–22.

19 MacIntyre DA, Chandiramani M, Lee YS, et al: The vaginal microbiome during pregnancy and the postpartum period in a European population. Sci Rep 2015;5:8988.
20 Romero R, Hassan SS, Gajer P, et al: The composition and stability of the vaginal microbiota of normal pregnant women is different from that of non-pregnant women. Microbiome 2014;2:4.
21 Fujiwara N, Tsuruda K, Iwamoto Y, et al: Significant increase of oral bacteria in the early pregnancy period in Japanese women. J Investig Clin Dent 2015, DOI: 10.1111/jicd.12189.
22 Goldenberg RL, Hauth JC, Andrews WW: Intrauterine infection and preterm delivery. N Engl J Med 2000;342:1500–1507.
23 Kovalovszki L, Villanyi Z, Pataki I, et al: Isolation of aerobic bacteria from the placenta. Acta Paediatr Acad Sci Hung 1982;23:357–360.
24 Lauder AP, Roche AM, Sherrill-Mix S, et al: Comparison of placenta samples with contamination controls does not provide evidence for a distinct placenta microbiota. Microbiome 2016;4:29.
25 Rautava S, Kainonen E, Salminen S, Isolauri E: Maternal probiotic supplementation during pregnancy and breast-feeding reduces the risk of eczema in the infant. J Allergy Clin Immunol 2012;130:1355–1360.
26 Kujovich JL: Thrombophilia and pregnancy complications. Am J Obstet Gynecol 2004;191:412–424.
27 Seong HS, Lee SE, Kang JH, et al: The frequency of microbial invasion of the amniotic cavity and histologic chorioamnionitis in women at term with intact membranes in the presence or absence of labor. Am J Obstet Gynecol 2008;199:375.e1–e5.
28 Mysorekar IU, Cao B: Microbiome in parturition and preterm birth. Semin Reprod Med 2014;32:50–55.
29 Hyman RW, Fukushima M, Jiang H, et al: Diversity of the vaginal microbiome correlates with preterm birth. Reprod Sci 2014;21:32–40.
30 Farr A, Kiss H, Holzer I, et al: Effect of asymptomatic vaginal colonization with *Candida albicans* on pregnancy outcome. Acta Obstet Gynecol Scand 2015;94:989–996.
31 Zi MY, Longo PL, Bueno-Silva B, Mayer MP: Mechanisms involved in the association between periodontitis and complications in pregnancy. Front Public Health 2014;2:290.
32 Offenbacher S, Boggess KS, Murtha AP, et al: Progressive periodontal disease and risk of very preterm delivery. Obstet Gynecol 2006;107:29–36.
33 ElAttar TM: Prostaglandin E2 in human gingiva in health and disease and its stimulation by female sex steroids. Prostaglandins 1976;11:331–341.
34 Kim J, Amar S: Periodontal disease and systemic conditions: a bidirectional relationship. Odontology 2006;94:10–21.

	Fetal life	Birth	Neonatal period and early infancy	
Source of microbes	Amniotic fluid? Maternal gut?	Birth canal Maternal gut	Modulation by human milk oligosaccharides Microbes in human milk?	
Gut microbiota characteristics	Low abundance of Enterobacteriaceae *Staphylococcus* *Streptococcus* *Lactobacillus*	*Lactobacillus* *Prevotella* *Sneathia* *Bacteroides* *Bifidobacterium*	Low diversity Dominated by bifidobacteria	
Potential perturbations	Maternal antibiotics? Maternal obesity?	Cesarean section - Low bacterial richness - Low bacterial diversity - Delayed colonization of Bacteroidetes	Neonatal antibiotics - Low bacterial diversity - Low bifidobacteria - Increase Proteobacteria	Formula feeding - Higher bacterial diversity - Fewer bifidobacteria

Fig. 1. The development of early gut microbiota.

microbes. During the past decades, it has become apparent that rather than mere cohabitance, our existence in the microbial world takes the form of mutually beneficial symbiosis. Indeed, except for erythrocytes, every human cell contains mitochondria, which are thought to originate from bacteria trapped inside our eukaryotic ancestors to form an essential part of our energy metabolism. Furthermore, our skin and mucosal surfaces harbor complex indigenous microbiota, which appears to be specific to both the anatomical site and the individual. The microbial community in the gastrointestinal tract and particularly the distal gut is currently most comprehensively understood. The predominant species of the gut microbiota are not frequently encountered in the environment, and it is therefore apparent that we obtain our indigenous microbes from other humans and, for the most part, from the mother. The vertical microbial transmission and colonization of the infant gut is a stepwise process (Fig. 1) disturbances of which may have deleterious consequences on health in infancy and beyond [1].

The contribution of commensal microbes for healthy immune and metabolic maturation has been the subject of rigorous scientific research over the past decade. It has become apparent that aberrant composition of the indigenous gut microbiota during early life is associated with the risk of developing immune-mediated and inflammatory disorders, including atopic disease, inflammatory bowel disease, type 1 diabetes mellitus, and obesity [reviewed in 1]. Perinatal and early-life factors, which may affect neonatal gut colonization, have also been linked to the risk of disease development (Table 1) [1]. Consequently, elucidating the origin and optimal composition of the gut microbiota during the first days, weeks, and months of life may be assumed to have significant clinical relevance.

19 MacIntyre DA, Chandiramani M, Lee YS, et al: The vaginal microbiome during pregnancy and the postpartum period in a European population. Sci Rep 2015;5:8988.
20 Romero R, Hassan SS, Gajer P, et al: The composition and stability of the vaginal microbiota of normal pregnant women is different from that of non-pregnant women. Microbiome 2014;2:4.
21 Fujiwara N, Tsuruda K, Iwamoto Y, et al: Significant increase of oral bacteria in the early pregnancy period in Japanese women. J Investig Clin Dent 2015, DOI: 10.1111/jicd.12189.
22 Goldenberg RL, Hauth JC, Andrews WW: Intrauterine infection and preterm delivery. N Engl J Med 2000;342:1500–1507.
23 Kovalovszki L, Villanyi Z, Pataki I, et al: Isolation of aerobic bacteria from the placenta. Acta Paediatr Acad Sci Hung 1982;23:357–360.
24 Lauder AP, Roche AM, Sherrill-Mix S, et al: Comparison of placenta samples with contamination controls does not provide evidence for a distinct placenta microbiota. Microbiome 2016;4:29.
25 Rautava S, Kainonen E, Salminen S, Isolauri E: Maternal probiotic supplementation during pregnancy and breast-feeding reduces the risk of eczema in the infant. J Allergy Clin Immunol 2012;130:1355–1360.
26 Kujovich JL: Thrombophilia and pregnancy complications. Am J Obstet Gynecol 2004; 191:412–424.
27 Seong HS, Lee SE, Kang JH, et al: The frequency of microbial invasion of the amniotic cavity and histologic chorioamnionitis in women at term with intact membranes in the presence or absence of labor. Am J Obstet Gynecol 2008;199:375.e1–e5.
28 Mysorekar IU, Cao B: Microbiome in parturition and preterm birth. Semin Reprod Med 2014;32:50–55.
29 Hyman RW, Fukushima M, Jiang H, et al: Diversity of the vaginal microbiome correlates with preterm birth. Reprod Sci 2014;21: 32–40.
30 Farr A, Kiss H, Holzer I, et al: Effect of asymptomatic vaginal colonization with *Candida albicans* on pregnancy outcome. Acta Obstet Gynecol Scand 2015;94:989–996.
31 Zi MY, Longo PL, Bueno-Silva B, Mayer MP: Mechanisms involved in the association between periodontitis and complications in pregnancy. Front Public Health 2014;2:290.
32 Offenbacher S, Boggess KS, Murtha AP, et al: Progressive periodontal disease and risk of very preterm delivery. Obstet Gynecol 2006; 107:29–36.
33 ElAttar TM: Prostaglandin E2 in human gingiva in health and disease and its stimulation by female sex steroids. Prostaglandins 1976; 11:331–341.
34 Kim J, Amar S: Periodontal disease and systemic conditions: a bidirectional relationship. Odontology 2006;94:10–21.

Isolauri E, Sherman PM, Walker WA (eds): Intestinal Microbiome: Functional Aspects in Health and Disease. Nestlé Nutr Inst Workshop Ser, vol 88, pp 11–21, (DOI: 10.1159/000455209)
Nestec Ltd., Vevey/S. Karger AG., Basel, © 2017

Microbial Composition of the Initial Colonization of Newborns

Samuli Rautava

Department of Pediatrics, Turku University Hospital, University of Turku, Turku, Finland

Abstract

Early-life interaction with indigenous intestinal microbes is a prerequisite for healthy immune and metabolic maturation. Human infants acquire their gut microbiota predominantly from the mother. A considerable inoculum of microbes is received by the neonate during vaginal delivery. Recent observations suggest that human gut colonization may be initiated prenatally by microbes in amniotic fluid, but the significance of this phenomenon remains unknown. After birth, neonatal gut colonization is guided by human milk factors, which selectively promote the growth of specific microbes, as well as by live microbes present in human milk. Aberrant gut colonization in early life has been associated with an increased risk of noncommunicable diseases in later life. Epidemiological and experimental studies suggest a causal relationship between early-life gut microbiota perturbations and disease risk. Perinatal antibiotic exposure, cesarean section delivery, postnatal antibiotic administration, and formula feeding, which may disrupt intestinal microecology, have been associated with disease development in later life. The modulation of gut microbiota in the perinatal period by pre- and probiotics, for example, may offer a means to reduce the risk of chronic diseases.

Introduction

At birth, the neonate enters a world inhabited by a myriad of microorganisms. While certain bacteria, viruses, and fungi represent a threat to health and well-being as potential pathogens, humans, among all other species on our planet, have evolved to live and thrive in an environment densely inhabited by

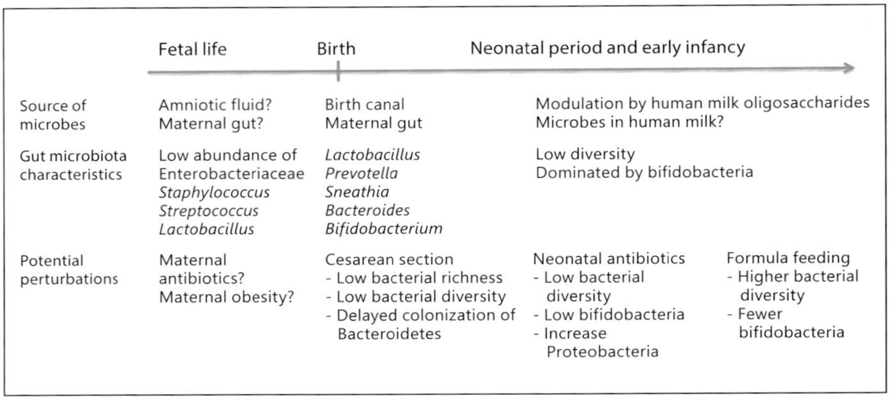

Fig. 1. The development of early gut microbiota.

microbes. During the past decades, it has become apparent that rather than mere cohabitance, our existence in the microbial world takes the form of mutually beneficial symbiosis. Indeed, except for erythrocytes, every human cell contains mitochondria, which are thought to originate from bacteria trapped inside our eukaryotic ancestors to form an essential part of our energy metabolism. Furthermore, our skin and mucosal surfaces harbor complex indigenous microbiota, which appears to be specific to both the anatomical site and the individual. The microbial community in the gastrointestinal tract and particularly the distal gut is currently most comprehensively understood. The predominant species of the gut microbiota are not frequently encountered in the environment, and it is therefore apparent that we obtain our indigenous microbes from other humans and, for the most part, from the mother. The vertical microbial transmission and colonization of the infant gut is a stepwise process (Fig. 1) disturbances of which may have deleterious consequences on health in infancy and beyond [1].

The contribution of commensal microbes for healthy immune and metabolic maturation has been the subject of rigorous scientific research over the past decade. It has become apparent that aberrant composition of the indigenous gut microbiota during early life is associated with the risk of developing immune-mediated and inflammatory disorders, including atopic disease, inflammatory bowel disease, type 1 diabetes mellitus, and obesity [reviewed in 1]. Perinatal and early-life factors, which may affect neonatal gut colonization, have also been linked to the risk of disease development (Table 1) [1]. Consequently, elucidating the origin and optimal composition of the gut microbiota during the first days, weeks, and months of life may be assumed to have significant clinical relevance.

Table 1. Association between early gut microbiota composition and the risk of diseases

	Characteristics of early gut microbiota preceding disease	Evidence of causality
Atopic disease	↓ Diversity ↓ Bifidobacteria ↓ Enterococci ↑ *Escherichia coli* ↑ *Clostridium difficile*	Experimental animal models ↑ After early AB ↑ After CS ↓ By probiotics
Obesity and overweight	↓ Bifidobacteria ↑ *Bacteroides fragilis*	Experimental animal models ↑ After AB ↑ After CS
Necrotizing enterocolitis	↓ Firmicutes ↑ Proteobacteria ↑ Clostridia	Experimental animal models ↑ After early AB ↓ By breast milk ↓ By probiotics
Infantile colic	↓ Diversity ↓ Bifidobacteria ↓ Lactobacilli ↑ Proteobacteria	↓ By probiotics

AB, antibiotic administration; CS, cesarean section.

Gut Colonization at Birth

The human neonate enters the extrauterine world through the birth canal, which is heavily populated with microbes. It is well established that maternal vaginal and intestinal microbes provide an important inoculum to the neonatal gut. Vaginal lactobacilli have been shown to transiently colonize the newborn intestine only to be replaced by bacteria from other maternal sources [2, 3]. The details on and the significance of this brief interaction with vaginal bacteria are not known. Based on studies comparing subjects born by vaginal or cesarean section (CS) delivery, it is evident that microbial contact during birth has a profound effect on gut colonization. In the immediate neonatal period, infants born by vaginal delivery harbor microbiota resembling that of the maternal vagina characterized by species belonging to *Lactobacillus*, *Prevotella*, and *Sneathia*, whereas subjects born by CS are colonized by bacteria typically found on the skin [3]. It is evident that the maternal gut is also an important source of colonizing microbes during vaginal delivery, since 72% of the early colonizers have been reported to match the species in the maternal gut in vaginally delivered newborns as compared to 41% in neonates born by CS [4]. The gut microbiota of vaginally delivered neonates are reportedly enriched by *Bacteroides*, *Bifidobacterium*,

Parabacteroides, and *Escherichia/Shigella* species in contrast to those born by CS, in whom bacteria typically encountered in the skin and mouth as well as the environment are frequently detected [4]. Later in infancy, infants born by CS reportedly display low bacterial richness and diversity [5] and delayed colonization by Bacteroidetes [6]. Differences in gut microbiota composition between vaginally and CS-delivered children have been detected until the age of 7 years [7].

There is compelling epidemiological evidence to suggest that birth by CS is associated with a significantly increased risk of obesity [8] and immune-mediated diseases such as asthma, inflammatory bowel disease, and arthritis in later life [9]. It is plausible that these detrimental long-term health effects of CS are at least partially attributable to aberrant gut colonization patterns, since the gut microbiota composition in early life has also been associated with the development of these disorders [1]. Still, it is conceivable that hormonal and immunomodulatory exposure during labor may also modulate disease risk in the offspring, or that confounding factors, such as maternal obesity, increase both the likelihood of CS as mode of birth and the risk of disease in the next generation. Meticulously conducted epidemiological studies and meta-analyses are needed to address these issues. It has recently been shown that the increase in the risk of asthma is particularly pronounced following CS conducted before rupture of membranes [10], which may possibly suggest a causal role for microbes in the process.

After the recognition of the significance of the microbial contact during delivery for the development of a healthy immune system and the risks associated with CS, an intriguing notion of inoculating maternal vaginal microbes to the neonate has been introduced [11]. The procedure is based on the general hypothesis that seeding vaginal microbes to the newborn infant directly following birth by CS might result in early colonization resembling that of vaginally delivered neonates and, consequently, reduce the risk of long-term health problems related to CS. The vaginal seeding procedure naturally also carries the risk of transmitting pathogenic microbes such as group B streptococci or the herpes simplex virus to the neonate, and measures need to be taken to minimize these risks. Furthermore, as discussed above, the neonate is also exposed to maternal intestinal microbes during vaginal delivery, and the significance of vaginal microbes for infant gut colonization remains largely unknown. Nonetheless, an interesting report from a preliminary study of 18 infants has recently been published [11]. In the 4 neonates inoculated with maternal vaginal microbes after CS delivery, the anal, oral, and skin microbiota of the infants at 1 month of age appeared to resemble that of vaginally delivered subjects more closely than infants born by CS without inoculation. Whether these changes in early colonization are associated with long-term differences in the indigenous microbiota or improved health outcomes remains to be determined by larger clinical trials.

Is the Fetal Gut Colonized by Microbes?

Several independent reports indicate that meconium, the first stool passed by the neonate but formed during fetal life, is not sterile [reviewed in 1]. Bacteria belonging predominantly to the phylum Firmicutes as well as species representing the genera *Enterobacterium, Bifidobacterium, Lactobacillus, Staphylococcus, Streptococcus,* and *Enterococcus* have been detected in low abundance in meconium using both traditional culture methods and culture-independent molecular techniques [12, 13]. The origin of the bacteria in meconium is currently not known. It is possible that the bacteria detected in meconium are not present in the intestine in utero but introduced at or after birth or even after passage. Nonetheless, data from experimental animal studies indicate that the fetal mouse gut harbors viable bacteria [14]. The intrauterine origin of the microbes in meconium is also corroborated by data indicating that the duration from rupture of membranes before delivery or the time from passage to analysis does not affect meconium bacterial counts [15].

It has been suggested that the bacteria in meconium are derived from amniotic fluid swallowed during fetal life [16]. This notion was originally suggested based on a comparison of microbial communities detected in meconium and previous reports on microbiota in amniotic fluid and at other sites [16]. We have recently provided data demonstrating similarities between meconium and amniotic fluid microbiota from the same mother-neonate pairs [13]. The amniotic fluid samples in the study were collected during sterile elective CS delivery to minimize the possibility of contamination. Several bacterial genera, including *Bacteroides, Lactobacillus, Prevotella,* and *Peptostreptococcus,* were detected in both amniotic fluid and meconium [13]. If the hypothesis of fetal gut colonization is further corroborated, the dogma of the sterile intrauterine compartment needs to be revised.

Small but detectable numbers of bacteria have been reported in the amniotic fluid and the pregnant and nonpregnant uterus outside the context of clinical infection using both conventional culture and molecular methods [1, 13]. A distinct microbiota dominated by enterobacteria has been reported in the placenta by Aagaard et al. [17]. Given the novelty of the hypothesis of a microbial community in the intrauterine compartment, the possibility of artifact or contamination needs to be carefully ruled out. False signals originating from the contamination of the reagents used in DNA purification may be problematic particularly when analyzing samples with very low microbial abundance. A recent study using quantitative PCR failed to detect consistent results distinguishing placenta samples from controls [18]. In contrast, we have published data corroborating the presence of microbes in both placenta and amniotic fluid using both conventional culture and denaturing gradient gel electrophoresis PCR and sequencing of the 16S rRNA gene [13]. To date, the bacterial genera detected in amniotic fluid or placenta include among others *Propionibacterium, Enterococcus, Staphylococcus, Citrobacter*, and *Lactobacillus* [13, 19]. Furthermore, intriguing experimental animal studies demonstrate that labeled *Enterococcus faecium* introduced into pregnant mice may be detected in the fetal gut [14]. These data suggest bacterial transfer from the mother to the fetal intestine, but our understanding of prenatal bacterial contact and its potential significance for subsequent gut colonization or later health is still virtually nonexistent.

Gut Microbiota in the Neonatal Period and Early Infancy

Human Milk as a Modulator of Gut Colonization

After birth, the most significant modulator of neonatal gut colonization is breast milk. In healthy newborns, initial neonatal gut microbiota characterized by *Escherichia coli,* enterococci, streptococci, and clostridia is rapidly followed by anaerobes including *Bifidobacterium* and *Bacteroides* species [20–22]. It is well established that the gut microbiota of breastfed infants is dominated by bifidobacteria [23, 24], which may be detectable already during the first days of life. In contrast, formula-fed infants harbor a more diverse gut microbiota [25] resembling that of older children. Breast milk contains a large array of nondigestable oligosaccharides (human milk oligosaccharides, HMO), one of the functions of which is to selectively promote the growth of specific intestinal bacteria and particularly bifidobacteria [reviewed in 26]. *Bifidobacterium longum* subspecies *infantis* is capable of utilizing a variety of HMOs [27] and, consequently, *B. longum* is almost universally detectable in the stool of breastfed infants from various geographical locations, including Northern Europe, Brazil, and Malawi [28, 29]. The role of HMOs in modulating gut colonization and human health is extensively reviewed elsewhere in this volume. It is of note, however, that in addition to HMOs, breast milk contains glycoproteins, which may also act as a source of selective substrates for specific bifidobacteria [30].

Human milk has been demonstrated to harbor a unique microbial community the composition of which is modulated by factors such as obesity, maternal immune-mediated disease, and mode of birth [reviewed in 31]. The origin of the bacteria in human milk remains elusive, but even the nonlactating mammary gland is reportedly colonized by bacteria [31]. It is likely that many of the microbes detected in milk originate from the skin. It is of note, however, that certain microbes typically detected in human milk, including lactic acid bacteria, are also characteristic of the human gut microbiota. Intestinal origin of milk microbes is suggested by observations according to which maternal intestinal microbes may be detected in peripheral blood immune cells and breast milk during lactation [32]. Based on these data, it has been suggested that maternal gut permeability is increased during lactation and that specific intestinal microbes are transported to the mammary gland by immune cells [32]. Consistently with this notion, the probiotic *Lactobacillus reuteri* has been detected in breast milk after maternal consumption in a clinical trial [33]. The physiological function of the bacteria in breast milk is not well understood, but it is possible that they function as a source of colonizers to the neonatal and infant gut. In accordance with this hypothesis, the neonatal gut microbiota shifts to bear resemblance to the microbial community in maternal milk during the first week of life [13], and there are data suggesting that breast milk microbes are transferred to the neonatal gut [34].

From an evolutionary point of view, the energy investment on HMOs on the mother's part, the profound impact of breastfeeding on early gut microbiota composition, and the unique predominance of bifidobacteria in the gut microbiota during breastfeeding are likely to provide a survival benefit for the infant. In line with this notion, epidemiological studies have linked disturbances in early gut microbiota composition and particularly reduced numbers of bifidobacteria to an increased risk of developing immune-mediated or inflammatory disorders such as atopic disease and obesity [reviewed in 1] (Table 1). Moreover, there are data to suggest that breastfeeding exerts a protective effect against a number of chronic, noncommunicable diseases [reviewed in 35]. It is possible but not proven that some of these beneficial effects of breastfeeding may result from the promotion of intestinal bifidobacteria.

Antibiotic Exposure

Exposure to antibiotics is known to exert a major effect on intestinal microecology and is relatively often followed by the development of diarrhea. It is alarming that antibiotic exposure in early life may also be associated with an increased risk of noncommunicable diseases, including asthma and obesity, in later life [reviewed in 1, 36]. While it is difficult to dissect the causal relationships between antibiotic exposure, the infections against which the antibiotics have been administered, and the development of chronic disease, based on both epidemiological and sophisticated experimental data, it has been suggested that aberrant gut microbiota composition resulting from early antibiotic exposure plays a causal role in the pathogenesis of obesity [reviewed in 36]. Given the significance of the neonatal period in gut colonization discussed above, it is of note that antibiotics are administered to 33–39% of mothers during delivery to prevent bacterial infection in the mother and the neonate [37, 38]. To date, relatively little is known about the effect of perinatal antibiotic exposure on gut colonization. A study based on 84 mother-infant pairs suggests that antibiotic prophylaxis administered because of maternal colonization with group B streptococci is associated with lower numbers of bifidobacteria detected by quantitative PCR in neonatal stool samples at the age of 7 days [39], but no differences were observed at the age of 30 days.

Early-onset neonatal sepsis is a devastating disease initially presenting with nonspecific symptoms or signs often followed by rapid deterioration. According to current guidelines, all infants with signs or symptoms suggesting sepsis as well as certain asymptomatic individuals with a high risk of infection based on the presence of factors such as chorioamnionitis should be subjected to empirical antibiotic therapy [36]. A large proportion of neonates (approximately 5%), therefore, receive broad-spectrum antibiotics during the first days of life [38].

Neonatal exposure to antibiotics has been reported to result in an increase in fecal Proteobacteria and particularly Enterobacteriaceae during the first weeks of life [40–42]. In addition, significant decreases in microbial diversity and in the abundance of *Bifidobacterium* have both been reported in neonates subjected to antibiotic interventions [40]. Our unpublished data suggest that gut microbiota perturbations caused by neonatal antibiotic exposure persist at least until the age of 6 months, but whether perinatal antibiotic exposure has an impact on the risk of disease in later life is currently not known.

Prematurity

Preterm newborns treated in neonatal intensive care units exhibit an aberrant gut microbiota composition in early life. Low diversity of the gut microbiota and delayed colonization with bifidobacteria have been associated with being born preterm [43, 44]. These disturbances may result directly from intestinal and immunologic immaturity. On the other hand, detrimental exposures including CS delivery, formula feeding, and early antibiotic exposure tend to cluster in preterm infants. Our unpublished observations suggest that while mode of birth, antibiotic exposure, and formula feeding, all have an impact on fecal bifidobacteria in late preterm infants, prematurity per se independently modulates *Bifidobacterium* colonization. Aberrant gut colonization in preterm infants has been suggested to be causally related to the risk of developing necrotizing enterocolitis [45] (Table 1), but whether the increase in metabolic risk factors associated with preterm birth is mediated by perturbations of early gut colonization remains unknown.

Conclusions

The composition of the early human gut microbiota has been associated with the development of noncommunicable diseases in later life [reviewed in 1]. Both reduced diversity and altered abundance of specific members of the intestinal ecosystem have been linked with various disorders ranging from atopic disease and obesity to infantile colic and necrotizing enterocolitis (Table 1). In addition, perinatal factors including CS delivery, antibiotic exposure, and formula feeding have been linked to both aberrant gut colonization patterns and an increased risk of chronic diseases later in childhood (Fig. 1; Table 1). Data from clinical and experimental studies may be interpreted to suggest that the link between early gut microbiota composition and disease risk may at least in part be causal, but our understanding of the interactions between the indigenous microbial community and ourselves, the host, are by no means complete. It is to be hoped that rigorous basic, translational, and clinical research will unravel these complex phenomena.

The potential causal role of early gut microbiota composition in the development of disease underscores the importance of supporting healthy gut colonization by reducing CS rates, prudent use of antibiotics, and promotion of breastfeeding. In addition, the intriguing possibility of reducing disease risk by modulating early microbial contact by prebiotics or probiotics deserves to be assessed. Thus far, the most convincing scientific evidence has been obtained from studies assessing the efficacy of early probiotic interventions in reducing the risk of atopic dermatitis [46] and necrotizing enterocolitis [47] in high-risk infants. Future studies will show whether prebiotics or probiotics are effective in the prevention of other chronic conditions, including obesity.

Disclosure Statement

Dr. Rautava's research has been funded by the Emil Aaltonen Foundation and the Finnish Foundation for Pediatric Research. He declares no conflict of interest, real or perceived.

References

1 Rautava S, Luoto R, Salminen S, Isolauri E: Microbial contact during pregnancy, intestinal colonization and human disease. Nat Rev Gastroenterol Hepatol 2012;9:565–576.

2 Matsumiya Y, Kato N, Watanabe K, Kato H: Molecular epidemiological study of vertical transmission of vaginal *Lactobacillus* species from mothers to newborn infants in Japanese, by arbitrarily primed polymerase chain reaction. J Infect Chemother 2002;8:43–49.

3 Dominguez-Bello MG, Costello EK, Contreras M, et al: Delivery mode shapes the acquisition and structure of the initial microbiota across multiple body habitats in newborns. Proc Natl Acad Sci U S A 2010;107:11971–11975.

4 Bäckhed F, Roswall J, Peng Y, et al: Dynamics and stabilization of the human gut microbiome during the first year of life. Cell Host Microbe 2015;17:690–703.

5 Azad MB, Konya T, Persaud RR, et al: Impact of maternal intrapartum antibiotics, method of birth and breastfeeding on gut microbiota during the first year of life: a prospective cohort study. BJOG 2016;123:983–993.

6 Jakobsson HE, Abrahamsson TR, Jenmalm MC, et al: Decreased gut microbiota diversity, delayed Bacteroidetes colonisation and reduced Th1 responses in infants delivered by caesarean section. Gut 2014;63:559–566.

7 Salminen S, Gibson GR, McCartney AL, Isolauri E: Influence of mode of delivery on gut microbiota composition in seven year old children. Gut 2004;53:1388–1389.

8 Kuhle S, Tong OS, Woolcott CG: Association between caesarean section and childhood obesity: a systematic review and meta-analysis. Obes Rev 2015;16:295–303.

9 Sevelsted A, Stokholm J, Bønnelykke K, Bisgaard H: Cesarean section and chronic immune disorders. Pediatrics 2015;135:e92–e98.

10 Sevelsted A, Stokholm J, Bisgaard H: Risk of asthma from cesarean delivery depends on membrane rupture. J Pediatr 2016;171:38–42.

11 Dominguez-Bello MG, De Jesus-Laboy KM, Shen N, et al: Partial restoration of the microbiota of cesarean-born infants via vaginal microbial transfer. Nat Med 2016;22:250–253.

12 Moles L, Gómez M, Heilig H, et al: Bacterial diversity in meconium of preterm neonates and evolution of their fecal microbiota during the first month of life. PLoS One 2013; 8:e66986.

13 Collado MC, Rautava S, Aakko J, et al: Human gut colonisation may be initiated in utero by distinct microbial communities in the placenta and amniotic fluid. Sci Rep 2016;6: 23129.

14 Jiménez E, Marín ML, Martín R, et al: Is meconium from healthy newborns actually sterile? Res Microbiol 2008;159:187–193.

15 Hansen R, Scott KP, Khan S, et al: First-pass meconium samples from healthy term vaginally-delivered neonates: an analysis of the microbiota. PLoS One 2015;10:e0133320.

16 Ardissone AN, de la Cruz DM, Davis-Richardson AG, et al: Meconium microbiome analysis identifies bacteria correlated with premature birth. PLoS One 2014;9:e90784.

17 Aagaard K, Ma J, Antony KM, et al: The placenta harbors a unique microbiome. Sci Transl Med 2014;6:237ra65.

18 Lauder AP, Roche AM, Sherrill-Mix S, et al: Comparison of placenta samples with contamination controls does not provide evidence for a distinct placenta microbiota. Microbiome 2016;4:29.

19 Zheng J, Xiao X, Zhang Q, et al: The placental microbiome varies in association with low birth weight in full-term neonates. Nutrients 2015;7:6924–6937.

20 Favier CF, de Vos WM, Akkermans AD: Development of bacterial and bifidobacterial communities in feces of newborn babies. Anaerobe 2003;9:219–229.

21 Solís G, de Los Reyes-Gavilan CG, Fernández N, et al: Establishment and development of lactic acid bacteria and bifidobacteria microbiota in breast-milk and the infant gut. Anaerobe 2010;16:307–310.

22 Jost T, Lacroix C, Braegger CP, Chassard C: New insights in gut microbiota establishment in healthy breast fed neonates. PLoS One 2012;7:e44595.

23 Harmsen HJ, Wildeboer-Veloo AC, Raangs GC, et al: Analysis of intestinal flora development in breast-fed and formula-fed infants by using molecular identification and detection methods. J Pediatr Gastroenterol Nutr 2000;30:61–67.

24 Roger LC, Costabile A, Holland DT, et al: Examination of faecal *Bifidobacterium* populations in breast- and formula-fed infants during the first 18 months of life. Microbiology 2010;156:3329–3341.
25 Azad MB, Konya T, Persaud RR, et al: Impact of maternal intrapartum antibiotics, method of birth and breastfeeding on gut microbiota during the first year of life: a prospective cohort study. BJOG 2016;123:983–993.
26 Bode L: Human milk oligosaccharides: every baby needs a sugar mama. Glycobiology 2012;22:1147–1162.
27 Underwood MA, German JB, Lebrilla CB, Mills DA: *Bifidobacterium longum* subspecies *infantis*: champion colonizer of the infant gut. Pediatr Res 2015;77:229–235.
28 Grześkowiak Ł, Collado MC, Mangani C, et al: Distinct gut microbiota in southeastern African and northern European infants. J Pediatr Gastroenterol Nutr 2012;54:812–816.
29 Grześkowiak Ł, Sales Teixeira TF, Bigonha SM, et al: Gut *Bifidobacterium* microbiota in one-month-old Brazilian newborns. Anaerobe 2015;35:54–58.
30 Karav S, Le Parc A, Leite Nobrega de Moura Bell JM, et al: Oligosaccharides released from milk glycoproteins are selective growth substrates for infant-associated bifidobacteria. Appl Environ Microbiol 2016;82:3622–3630.
31 Collado MC, Rautava S, Isolauri E, Salminen S: Gut microbiota – source of novel tools to reduce the risk of human disease? Pediatr Res 2015;77:182–188.
32 Perez PF, Doré J, Leclerc M, et al: Bacterial imprinting of the neonatal immune system: lessons from maternal cells? Pediatrics 2007; 119:e724–e732.
33 Abrahamsson TR, Sinkiewicz G, Jakobsson T, et al: Probiotic lactobacilli in breast milk and infant stool in relation to oral intake during the first year of life. J Pediatr Gastroenterol Nutr 2009;49:349–354.
34 Jost T, Lacroix C, Braegger CP, et al: Vertical mother-neonate transfer of maternal gut bacteria via breastfeeding. Environ Microbiol 2014;16:2891–2904.
35 Rautava S, Walker WA: Academy of Breastfeeding Medicine founder's lecture 2008: breastfeeding – an extrauterine link between mother and child. Breastfeed Med 2009;4: 3–10.
36 Turta O, Rautava S: Antibiotics, obesity and the link to microbes – what are we doing to our children? BMC Med 2016;14:57.
37 Stokholm J, Schjørring S, Pedersen L, et al: Prevalence and predictors of antibiotic administration during pregnancy and birth. PLoS One 2013;8:e82932.
38 Persaud RR, Azad MB, Chari RS, et al: Perinatal antibiotic exposure of neonates in Canada and associated risk factors: a population-based study. J Matern Fetal Neonatal Med 2015;28:1190–1195.
39 Corvaglia L, Tonti G, Martini S, et al: Influence of intrapartum antibiotic prophylaxis for group B *Streptococcus* on gut microbiota in the first month of life. J Pediatr Gastroenterol Nutr 2016;62:304–308.
40 Fouhy F, Guinane CM, Hussey S, et al: High-throughput sequencing reveals the incomplete, short-term recovery of infant gut microbiota following parenteral antibiotic treatment with ampicillin and gentamicin. Antimicrob Agents Chemother 2012;56: 5811–5820.
41 Arboleya S, Sánchez B, Milani C, et al: Intestinal microbiota development in preterm neonates and effect of perinatal antibiotics. J Pediatr 2015;166:538–544.
42 Greenwood C, Morrow AL, Lagomarcino AJ, et al: Early empiric antibiotic use in preterm infants is associated with lower bacterial diversity and higher relative abundance of Enterobacter. J Pediatr 2014;165:23–29.
43 Magne F, Abély M, Boyer F, et al: Low species diversity and high interindividual variability in faeces of preterm infants as revealed by sequences of 16S rRNA genes and PCR-temporal temperature gradient gel electrophoresis profiles. FEMS Microbiol Ecol 2006;57: 128–138.
44 Arboleya S, Binetti A, Salazar N, et al: Establishment and development of intestinal microbiota in preterm neonates. FEMS Microbiol Ecol 2012;79:763–772.
45 Neu J, Walker W: Necrotizing enterocolitis. N Engl J Med 2011;364:255–264.
46 Isolauri E, Rautava S, Salminen S: Probiotics in the development and treatment of allergic disease. Gastroenterol Clin North Am 2012; 41:747–762.
47 AlFaleh K, Anabrees J: Probiotics for prevention of necrotizing enterocolitis in preterm infants. Cochrane Database Syst Rev 2014; 4:CD005496.

Isolauri E, Sherman PM, Walker WA (eds): Intestinal Microbiome: Functional Aspects in Health and Disease. Nestlé Nutr Inst Workshop Ser, vol 88, pp 23–33, (DOI: 10.1159/000455210)
Nestec Ltd., Vevey/S. Karger AG., Basel, © 2017

Bacterial Colonization of the Newborn Gut, Immune Development, and Prevention of Disease

W. Allan Walker

Mucosal Immunology and Biology Research Center, MassGeneral Hospital for Children, Charlestown, MA, and Division of Nutrition, Harvard Medical School, Boston, MA, USA

Abstract

We now know that the fetus does not reside in a sterile intrauterine environment but is exposed to commensal bacteria from the maternal gut which cross the placenta and infiltrate the amniotic fluid. This exposure to colonizing bacteria continues at birth and during the first year of life, and it has a profound influence on lifelong health. Why is this important? Cross talk with colonizing bacteria in the developing neonatal intestine helps in the initial adaptation of the infant to extrauterine life, particularly in acquiring immune homeostasis, and provides protection against disease expression (e.g., allergy, autoimmune disease, and obesity) later in life. Colonizing intestinal bacteria are critical to the development of host defense during the neonatal period. Disrupted colonization (dysbiosis) due to cesarean section delivery, perinatal antibiotics, or premature delivery may adversely affect the development of host defense mechanisms in the gut and predispose to inflammation leading to increased susceptibility to disease later in life. Clinical evidence suggests that babies born by cesarean section have higher incidence rates of allergy, type 1 diabetes, and obesity. Infants given repeated antibiotic regimens are more likely to have asthma as adolescents. This observation helps to explain the disease paradigm shift in children from developed countries.

Introduction

In the last half century, the disease burden in developed countries has shifted from a predominately infectious to an immune basis [1]. For example, there has been a striking increase in allergic and autoimmune diseases. This shift and increase in disease has been attributed to the nature of initial bacterial colonization of the newborn intestine, a revision of the so-called "hygiene hypothesis" [2]. During the first 2 years of life, the infant establishes a complete colonization of the gastrointestinal tract that remains as a microbial signature throughout his life. The initial colonization process occurs in stages and has its greatest fluctuations in the early few months of life. During the same neonatal period, the newborn infant develops appropriate intestinal host defenses to protect him from infectious and immune-mediated diseases. Since intestinal bacteria influence gut metabolic and immunologic function, the fluctuations in bacterial colonization at the time when immune homeostasis is developing has a profound effect on the infant's general health and the prevention of disease expression later in life.

An example of this process is the development of immune tolerance. Immune tolerance to innocuous antigens and commensal bacteria is the absence of a systemic immune response to their stimulus and thus an absence of autoimmune disease states. Oral tolerance develops only with bacterial colonization [3] which also defines appropriate immunologic responses to stimuli including the nature of the T-helper cell subset response and other immunologic cellular subsets [4]. As new studies are reported regarding the association between intestinal colonization and host defense, we have come to appreciate the importance of appropriate initial colonization and immune homeostasis.

Normal Intestinal Colonization – Symbiosis

We now know that the human fetus does not reside in a sterile environment [5]. Experimental and clinical evidence exists to suggest that the human fetus is exposed to bacteria in utero. Microbiota have been identified in the placenta, amniotic fluid, and meconium of full-term, vaginally delivered, healthy newborns suggesting that exposure to microbes in utero occurs under normal gestational conditions. Furthermore, the nature of the pregnant mother's environment (e.g., weight gain or exposure to infection) during gestation can impact on fetal exposure to microorganisms. Details of these processes are covered by other authors/speakers in this symposium.

Normal intestinal bacterial colonization leading to immune homeostasis and the absence of disease occurs in full-term, vaginally delivered newborns not exposed to perinatal antibiotics. These infants exhibit so-called "pioneer" bacteria which have a specific effect on the normal development of intestinal host defense including oral tolerance [6]. Normal colonization occurs in various phases over the first 18 months to 2 years of life (Table 1). Phase 1, the most important phase, occurs with the ingestion of a healthy bolus of maternal vaginal/colonic bacteria

Table 1. Phases of normal (symbiotic) initial bacterial colonization

Phase 0
Partial colonization in the intrauterine environment
Phase 1
Acquire maternal vaginal/colonic microbiota (full-term vaginal delivery)
Phase 2
Introduction of oral feedings (breast milk vs. formula)
Phase 3
Weaning to solid foods
Phase 4
Acquire complete mature colonization (12–18 months) (>1,000 different species)

as the vaginally delivered, partially intrauterine-colonized infant passes through the birth canal. Phase 2 is the stimulus of oral feeding on bacterial proliferation. The nature of initial oral feeding (breast milk vs. formula) is a major determinant of normal colonization. Phase 3 occurs when the infant is weaned to complementary solid foods. By 18 months to 2 years of life, a mature intestinal colonization signature exists which is unique to that child throughout his life. Final colonization consists of microbiota (1,013/mL intestinal content) residing principally in the distal small intestine and colon as anaerobic bacteria. The nature of colonizing bacteria is very diverse, consisting of over 2,000 different species. Although genetics contributes to the nature of colonizing bacteria, environmental factors are very important and will be considered in a separate section.

Dietary Influence on Colonization

Although other environmental factors (antibiotics, vaccinations, and hygienic conditions) are very important determinants in intestinal bacterial colonization, the most important environmental factor is diet. Diet is particularly important in infancy when the microbial colonizing signature is evolving and has its major influence on gastrointestinal host defense. Breastfed infants have strikingly different microbiota than formula-fed infants. Components of breast milk, including oligosaccharides, stimulate so-called "pioneer" bacteria which can influence intestinal function such as an increase in polymeric IgA and a decrease in the intestinal IL-6 inflammatory response [7]. A new area of research has developed to determine what other protective factors in breast milk (e.g., lactoferrin, transforming growth factor-β, or fatty acids) influence initial bacterial colonization. In a recent experimental study, for example, the absence of breast milk-induced polymeric IgA given to newborn rodent pups affects the intestinal microbiota and predisposes to a greater access of gram-positive organisms to the mucosal barrier [8]. In addition, intestinal bacteria induced by breastfeeding can stimulate enterocyte genes that both promote intestinal development and immune protection [9]. Furthermore, recent studies have suggested that breast milk has its own microbiome consisting in part of commensal bacteria found in mother's intestinal tract [10]. To what extent the ingestion of breast milk bacteria influence the ultimate composition of the infant's intestinal microbiota has not yet been determined.

Other studies have suggested that diet can influence gut colonization at various periods throughout life. An experimental study has shown that when common probiotic organisms (bifidobacteria or lactobacilli) are grown in either high-carbohydrate-, (saturated and unsaturated) fat-, or protein-containing media, a differential proliferation of the probiotic bacteria can occur as well as a differential stimulation of specific bacterial genes [11]. In addition, a recent study comparing the microbiome of children living in a primitive village in Africa with that of children in a city in a developed country (Florence, Italy) showed a striking difference in their microbiomes suggesting that diet (a complex carbohydrate diet with no animal fat or protein [Africa] versus a standard Western diet including processed foods [Italy]) had a strong influence on the composition of intestinal colonizing bacteria [12]. Although not specifically studied, it is known that the disease burden between these 2 patient populations differs dramatically suggesting that the influence of diet on microbiome content may in turn impact on long-term health. Finally, a recent large clinical study suggested that long-term modifications in diet (carbohydrate vs. fat) affect [5] the individual's enterotype (functional clusters of bacteria) expression of intestinal bacteria [13].

Immunologic Consequences of Normal Colonization

Evidence exists that during a full-term pregnancy components of mucosal immune function in the fetuses can develop. However, for these intestinal defense components to be activated, the intestine must first be stimulated by initial bacterial colonization with appropriate commensal bacteria [14] (Fig. 1). In a like manner, other host defense functions that provide an intact mucosal barrier such as tight junctions, microfold cells, or glycocalyx to prevent the uptake of pathogens and noxious antigens are stimulated by the initial colonization process [15]. Accordingly, an appropriate initial intestinal colonization is necessary for immunologic adaptation of the neonate to the extrauterine environment (Table 2).

Initial colonization is necessary for both innate and adaptive immune function. Colonizing bacteria stimulate enterocytes and mucosal lymphoid cells

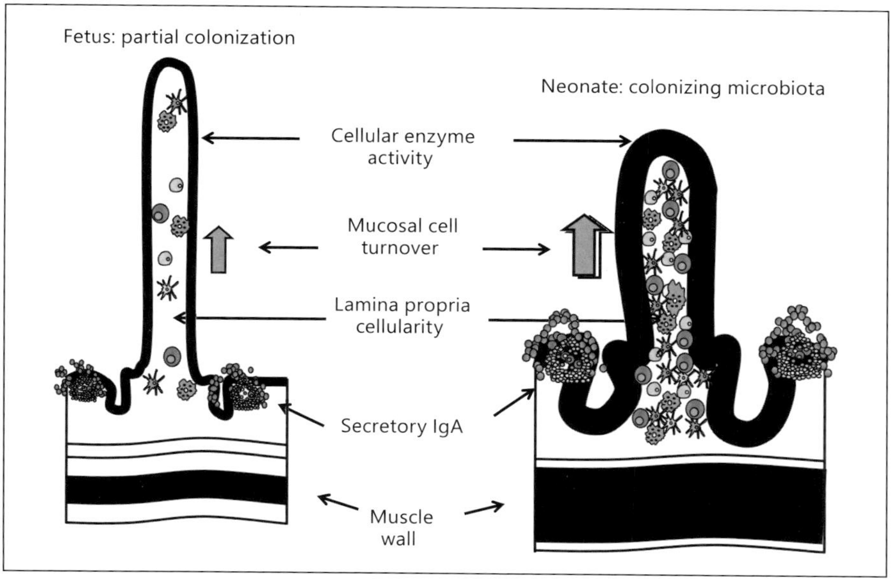

Fig. 1. The influence of colonization on intestinal function (intra- versus extrauterine gut) is depicted as a schematic cross section of the small intestine of a human fetus in utero versus that of a newborn infant. The fetal intestine appears thin and exhibits a slow epithelial proliferation rate with a paucity of gut-associated lymphoid tissue (GALT), whereas the infant intestine manifests a robust, diverse epithelium with a fast turnover rate and abundant GALT elements. Reprinted from Walker [14] with permission.

Table 2. Microbial colonization and immunologic adaptation to the extrauterine environment

Protective enterocyte barrier functions
Innate immune responses
Adaptive immune responses
Polymeric IgA secretion
Balanced T-helper cell responses
Oral tolerance

(e.g., macrophages and lymphocytes) to react to pathogens attempting to cross the mucosal barrier by evoking an inflammatory response. These reactions are mediated by pattern recognition receptors such as toll-like receptors expressed on these cells to interact with the pathogens initiating an inflammatory (IL-6 or IL-8) response to prevent penetration. Colonizing bacteria stimulate intestinal cells to upregulate signaling molecules in order to react to potential penetration. However, over time with repeated stimulation, these intestinal cells become tolerant to exposure in order to prevent chronic

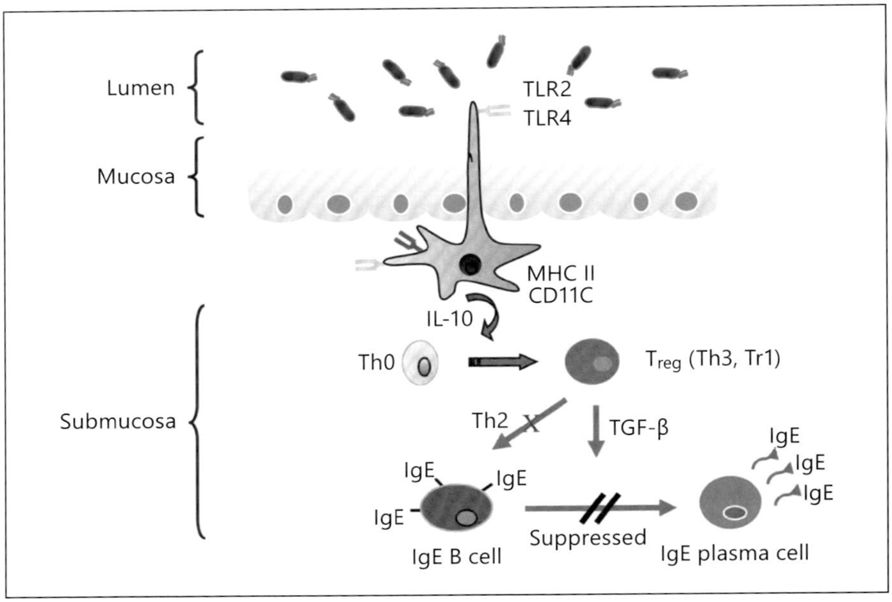

Fig. 2. Physiologic immune response to intestinal antigens is shown as a schematic representation of oral tolerance induction by gut microbiota. In the intestinal lumen, gut microbiota activates dendritic cells via the TLR2/TLR4 signaling pathways. Activated dendritic cells cause maturation of Th0 to subsets (Th3, Tr1) of T_{reg} cells via the release of IL-10 to stimulate TGF-β release and thereby suppress humoral IgE production. Reprinted from Walker [14] with permission.

inflammation of the intestine [16] leading to diseases such as inflammatory bowel diseases.

In a like manner, colonizing bacteria prime T-helper cells subsets (Th1, Th2, Th17, and T_{reg}) to activate a balanced immunologic response and to evoke on intestinal immune homeostasis rather than inflammation [17]. These stimulated T-helper cells produce a balanced humoral and cellular immune response including an appropriate T-regulatory reaction leading to immune tolerance.

A major component of intestinal protective function is the capacity to develop oral tolerance to commensal bacteria and innocuous antigens. Oral tolerance occurs when repeated exposures to oral antigens stimulate mucosal T-regulatory cells to release cytokines such as IL-10 and TGF-β that downregulate both humoral and cellular immune responses (Fig. 2). Oral tolerance must exist to prevent inappropriate inflammatory reactions to these benign antigens and thus prevent inflammatory disease. The increase in immune-mediated diseases in developed countries is attributed to a lack of oral tolerance development. A normal, balanced, initial colonization during the newborn period is necessary to activate oral tolerance and to prevent the expression of allergic and other immune-mediated diseases later in life [18]. Thus, normal initial colonization of the neonatal gastrointestinal tract is necessary for the development of appropriate intestinal immunoprotective function and the prevention of disease.

Dysbiosis

Dysbiosis, the abnormal colonization of the intestine with less species diversity and altered phyla, can unfortunately commonly occur with the initial colonization of the newborn intestine [19]. Thus, dysbiosis provides colonizing bacteria which either fail to activate the needed immunoprotective function or actually stimulate a distinct immune response (an imbalance in lymphocytes or the upregulation of immune cells which favor inflammation). As a result, the developing intestine established abnormal immunologic responses to stimuli leading to the expression of chronic disease later in life. Details of dysbiosis in the newborn period will be discussed in detail by other authors/speakers. As stated, dysbiotic colonization can disrupt the normal development of intestinal host defenses which may result in the expression of immune-mediated diseases (allergy, type 1 diabetes, or celiac disease) later in life. Dysbiosis is thought to be a major contributor to the observed shift in the disease paradigm within developed countries over the last several decades. Although there is a genetic component to dysbiosis in newborn colonization, environmental factors are thought to be a major contributing factor. Lifestyle factors such as diet and stress can affect the nature of colonizing bacteria. In addition, the nature of initial exposure to microbiota in the perinatal period (birth by cesarean section or prolonged hospitalization in the neonatal intensive care unit) can also contribute. Furthermore, medical practices such as the use of antibiotics, excessive vaccination, and excessive cleanliness can disrupt the initial colonizing process. All these circumstances disrupt the appropriate development of intestinal homeostasis and favor disease processes which occur with inflammation.

The process of abnormal colonization differs strikingly from the normal process (Table 3). As a result of premature delivery, birth by cesarean section, and the use of perinatal antibiotics, initial colonization results in a sparse, inadequate phase 1 of the colonization process. Despite the stimulus of oral feeding and weaning to solid foods, the complete colonization of the intestine under these conditions is delayed until 4–6 years of life. During that time period, the infant is more susceptible to both infectious and immune-mediated diseases. Microbial dysbiosis as a result of abnormal colonization has been associated with an increased incidence of chronic diseases later in life. A scientific

Table 3. Phases of abnormal initial bacterial colonization (dysbiosis[1])

Phase 1
Sparse, inadequate colonization due to:
Premature delivery
Cesarean section delivery
Use of perinatal antibiotics
Phases 2, 3
Introduction of oral feeding and weaning results in slight modifications
Phase 4
Delayed, incomplete initial colonization until 4–6 years

[1] More susceptible to pathogens and immune-mediated diseases, e.g. allergic diseases.

study done on newborn rat pups given low-dose antibiotics has been attributed to their increase in weight gain leading to obesity when placed on a high saturated fat diet later in life [20]. This association occurs despite a return to normal intestinal microbiota after the initial exposure to antibiotics underscoring the importance of disrupted dysbiotic colonization early in life on long-term expression of disease. This same observation has been made clinically when mothers gain excessive weight during pregnancy resulting in disruption of their intestinal microbiota, which in turn is passed to their infants at the time of birth, predisposing these infants to excessive weight gain and eventual obesity [21]. Infants born by cesarean section have an increased incidence of allergic diseases such as asthma during adolescence as well as other autoimmune diseases. The same observation has been made with newborns receiving perinatal antibiotics. Thus, early dysbiosis may have profound effects on health later in life.

We have studied the pathogenesis of necrotizing enterocolitis (NEC) for many years. Using ex vivo models of human fetal intestine and primary enterocytes from NEC patients, we have shown that initial commensal colonizing bacteria evoke an inflammatory response as opposed to oral tolerance in immature enterocytes as a result of underdeveloped innate inflammatory genetic pathways [22]. Others have shown that the composition of microbiota in NEC patients differs from that of age-related premature infants in the absence of NEC. A recent study from this laboratory [23] indicated that the more immature the intestine of prematures (e.g. infants <1,000 g) the more dysbiotic is the colonizing microbiome indicating that intestinal immaturity may influence intestinal colonization. This observation suggests that the basis for NEC in premature infants appears to be related to a dysbiotic colonization as well as an immature, proinflammatory response to commensal bacteria.

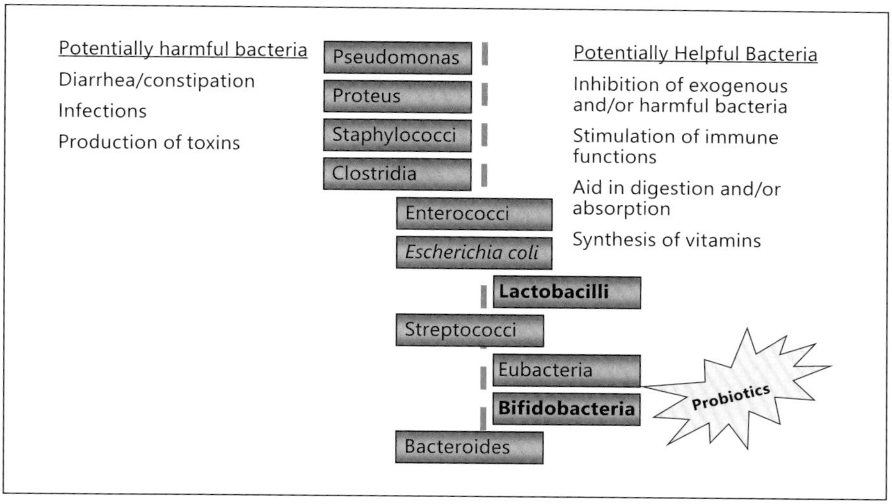

Fig. 3. Intestinal microbiota restoration with probiotics. Under conditions of dysbiosis, an imbalance exists between potentially harmful and helpful bacteria. Probiotics may help to restore the dysbiosis to a symbiotic state.

Use of Probiotics

The use of probiotics to correct dysbiotic colonization (Fig. 3) will be discussed by other authors/speakers. The intent of this section is to briefly suggest that probiotics have been effective in partially restoring symbiosis to a dysbiotic colonization process. In our studies with breast milk, we have shown that compared to formula-fed premature infants those fed mother's expressed breast milk have a microbiota which favors anti-inflammation over inflammation. This may be an explanation for the protective effect against NEC seen in premature infants given expressed breast milk. Other studies suggest that specific probiotics (e.g., *Bifidobacterium infantis*) may preferentially inhibit inflammation in premature infants. We have just published an observation to suggest that unique to the immature enterocyte response of those exposed to *B. infantis* secretions to decrease inflammation is the use of TLR4 expressed on the surface of these enterocytes [24]. Probiotics have also been effectively used to reduce the expression of atopic dermatitis in allergy-prone infants when given in later stages of pregnancy and during lactation in mothers with a history of allergy [25] (to be discussed by other authors/speakers).

This area of investigation requires additional clinical and scientific studies before recommendations for the routine management of premature infants can be made.

Summary and Conclusions

In this review, a case has been made for the importance of normal initial colonization of the newborn intestine for an optimum adaptation of the infant to the extrauterine environment. Evidence is provided that colonizing bacteria activate the appropriate expression of intestinal defenses including components of the mucosal barrier as well as both innate and adaptive immune responses including oral tolerance. Normal colonization is dependent on both genetic and environmental factors, especially the influence of diet on the composition of intestinal microbiota. This observation is particularly true of breast feeding as the initial source of oral feeding. Factors in breast milk affect the composition of intestinal microbiota by stimulating "pioneer" bacteria which are essential in the activation of intestinal immune defenses such as polymeric IgA production. Disruption of normal colonization, dysbiosis, caused by prematurity, cesarean section, or the use of perinatal antibiotics can adversely affect the interaction of symbiotic commensals and host defense predisposing to disease expression, e.g., allergy, later in life. Thus, the dysbiotic effect on disease expression may be reversed by the use of probiotics. However, additional clinical studies are required.

Disclosure Statement

The author has no conflict of interest.

References

1 Bach JF: The effect of infections on susceptibility to autoimmune and allergic diseases. N Engl J Med 2002;347:911–920.

2 Guarner F, Bourdet-Sicardf R, Brandtzaeg P, et al: Mechanisms of disease: the hygiene hypothesis revisited. Nat Clin Pract Gastroenterol Hepatol 2006;3:275–284.

3 Sudo N, Sawamura S, Tanaka K, Aiba Y, Kubo C, Koga Y: The requirement of intestinal bacterial flora for the development of an IgE production system fully susceptible to oral tolerance induction. J Immunol 1997; 159:1739–1745.

4 Kaplan JL, Shi H, Walker WA: The role of microbes in developmental immunologic programming. Pediatr Res 2011;69:465–472.

5 Donnet-Hughes A, Schriffin E, Walker WA: Protective properties of human milk and bacterial colonization of the neonatal gut; in Duggan C, Koletzko B, Watkins J, Walker WA (eds): Nutrition in Pediatrics – Basic Science and Clinical Applications, ed 5. New Haven, Chinese Publications, 2015, chapt 30, pp 150–165.

6 Jost T, Lacroix C, Braegger C, et al: New insights into gut microbiota establishment in healthy breast fed neonates. PLoS One 2012; 7:e44595.

7 Bode L: Human milk oligosaccharides: every baby needs a sugar mama. Glycobiology 2012;22:1147–1162.

8 Rogier EW, Frantz AI, Bruno MEC, et al: Secretory antibodies in breast milk promote long-term intestinal homeostasis by regulating the gut microbiota and host gene expression. Proc Natl Acad Sci U S A 2014;111: 3074–3079.

9 Schwartz S, Friedberg I, Ivanov IV, et al: A metagenomic study of diet-dependent interaction between gut microbiota and host in infants reveals differences in immune response. Genome Biol 2012;13:r32.

10 Jeurink PV, van Bergenhenegouwen J, Jiménez E, et al: Human milk: a source of more life than we imagine. Benef Microbes 2013;4: 17–30.

11 Faith JJ, McNulty NP, Rey FE, et al: Predicting a human gut microbiota's response to diet in gnotobiotic mice. Science 2011;333: 101–104.

12 DeFilippo C, Cavalieri D, DiPaola M, et al: Impact of diet in shaping gut microbiota revealed by a comparative study in children from Europe and rural Africa. Proc Natl Acad Sci U S A 2010;107:14691–14696.

13 Wu GD, Chen J, Hoffman C, et al: Linking long-term dietary patterns with gut microbial enterotypes. Science 2011;334:105–108.

14 Walker WA: Initial intestinal colonization in the human infant and immune homeostasis. Ann Nutr Metab 2013;63(suppl 2):8–15.

15 Artis D: Epithelial-cell recognition of commensal bacteria and maintenance of immune homeostasis in the gut. Nat Rev Immunol 2008;8:411–420.

16 Otte JM, Cario E, Podolsky DK: Mechanism of cross hyporesponsiveness to toll-like receptor bacterial ligands in intestinal epithelial cells. Gastroenterology 2004;126:1054–1070.

17 Hooper LV, Littman DR, Macpherson AJ: Interactions between the microbiota and the immune system. Science 2012;336:1268–1273.

18 Weng M, Walker WA: The role of gut microbiota in programming the immune phenotype. J Dev Orig Health Dis 2013;4:203–214.

19 Rautava S, Luoto R, Salminen S, et al: Microbial contact during pregnancy, intestinal colonization and human disease. Nat Rev Gastroenterol Hepatol 2012;9:565–576.

20 Blaser M: Antibiotic overuse: stop killing of beneficial bacteria. Nature 2011;476:393–394.

21 Baker JL, Michaelsen KF, Rasmussen KM, Sorensen TIA: Maternal prepregnant body mass index, duration of breastfeeding, and timing of complementary food introduction are associated with infant weight gain. Am J Clin Nutr 2004;80:1579–1588.

22 Claud EC, Lu L, Anton PM, et al: Developmentally regulated IκB expression in intestinal epithelium and susceptibility to flagellin-induced inflammation. Proc Natl Acad Sci U S A 2004;101:7404–7408.

23 Zhou Y, Shan G, Sodergren E, et al: Longitudinal analysis of premature infant intestinal microbiome prior to necrotizing enterocolitis: a case-control study. PLoS One 2015; 10:e0118632.

24 Meng D, Zhu W, Shi HN, et al: The toll-like receptor-4 in human and mouse colonic epithelium is developmentally regulated: a possible role in necrotizing enterocolitis. Pediatr Res 2015;77:416–424.

25 Kalliomäki M, Salminen S, Arvilommi H, et al: Probiotics in primary prevention of atopic disease: a randomized placebo-controlled trial. Lancet 2001;357:1076–1079.

Isolauri E, Sherman PM, Walker WA (eds): Intestinal Microbiome: Functional Aspects in Health and Disease. Nestlé Nutr Inst Workshop Ser, vol 88, pp 35–44, (DOI: 10.1159/000455211)

Epigenetics in Gastrointestinal Health and Disease: Spotlight on DNA Methylation in the Intestinal Epithelium

Matthias Zilbauer · Judith Kraiczy

Department of Paediatrics, University of Cambridge, Addenbrooke's Hospital, Cambridge, UK

Abstract

Epigenetics can be defined as stable, potentially heritable changes in cellular phenotype caused by mechanisms other than alterations in the underlying DNA sequence. DNA methylation is amongst the most intensely studied epigenetic mechanisms and has been shown to play a major role in regulating fundamental aspects of cell biology including cellular differentiation, organ development, and cell type-specific gene expression. Importantly, it is becoming increasingly clear that epigenetic mechanisms operate at the interface between the genetic code and our environment and are able to mediate environmental changes into stable phenotypic alterations. Given existing evidence supporting the important effects of environmental factors (e.g., diet, nutrition, and infections) on human health, epigenetic mechanisms provide a plausible mechanistic framework for the development of many multifactorial diseases including inflammatory bowel disease (IBD). Impaired function of the intestinal epithelium has been implicated in IBD pathogenesis, yet underlying mechanisms remain ill defined. The work of our group focuses on investigating the role of DNA methylation in regulating cellular function of the human intestinal epithelium during gastrointestinal health and IBD. In addition to performing an analysis of primary human intestinal epithelium, we utilize human intestinal organoid culture systems allowing us to perform functional analysis in a patient-derived ex vivo model.

Introduction

The basic concept of epigenetics was first proposed by Conrad Hall Waddington [1] in 1942. As a developmental biologist, he coined the term "epigenetic landscape" describing the way in which genes interact with the environment to ultimately produce a phenotype. Today, epigenetics can be defined as molecular mechanism(s) capable of changing an organism's phenotype without altering the underlying DNA sequence. These changes are potentially heritable, allowing epigenetic marks to be passed on to daughter cells during mitosis and potentially even across generations [2]. Importantly, it is becoming increasingly clear that epigenetic mechanisms operate at the interface between the human genome and our environment and are capable of translating external stimuli into phenotypic cellular changes.

The human intestinal tract represents a fascinating example for the capability of adapting to the environment. Following in utero development, the intestinal mucosa is being colonized postnatally by a vast number and variety of microbes while being exposed to a multitude of increasingly complex nutrients. Interestingly, it is well established that exposure to these environmental factors is critical for the physiological and functional development of the gastrointestinal (GI) tract. Conversely, alterations in these processes, possibly as a result of changes in our environment, are increasingly being recognized as major factors contributing to the development of GI-related diseases such as necrotizing enterocolitis and inflammatory bowel disease (IBD).

The intestinal epithelium, as the single cell layer separating the host from its environment, has long been recognized as playing a major role in orchestrating homeostasis in the GI tract. The close contact and constant exposure of the epithelium to the intestinal microbiota, nutrients as well as potential toxins, make it an ideal cell type to investigate the role of epigenetic mechanisms in regulating cellular function during physiological gut development. Moreover, substantial evidence supports a key role of the intestinal epithelium in GI pathology, further expanding the relevance of this exciting new field of biomedical research.

In the following, we provide a brief introduction to the basic molecular principles of epigenetics and highlight some of the existing evidence for the role of epigenetic mechanisms in GI health and disease with a particular focus on the role of DNA methylation in the intestinal epithelium. Lastly, we will introduce human intestinal epithelial organoids as emerging models to study intestinal epithelial cell biology including epigenetic mechanisms in health and disease.

Epigenetics – Basic Principles

Currently, the main epigenetic mechanisms known to be operative in mammals are DNA methylation and hydroxymethylation, expression of noncoding RNAs, and posttranslational modifications of histone proteins.

The latter occurs primarily on histone tails (N-termini) and includes acetylation, methylation, and phosphorylation for example [3]. Posttranslational modifications of histones alter the chromatin state, which is defined as a complex of DNA, RNA, and proteins, and thereby influence gene transcription and ultimately cellular function. Non-protein-coding RNAs, such as microRNAs, are short RNA sequences (i.e. 20–23 nucleotides), which regulate gene transcription by preventing the translation of mRNA into protein by binding to a short complementary region. This binding process can activate a microRNA-induced silencing complex including endoribonuclease, an enzyme capable of cleaving double-stranded RNA, and, therefore, prevent translation of mRNA into protein.

Lastly, DNA methylation is amongst the most extensively studied epigenetic mechanisms and occurs primarily in the 5′ position of the pyrimidine ring of cytosines in the context of CpG dinucleotides (5-methylcytosine). The majority of CpGs in the human genome are known to be methylated, with the major exception being CpG-rich areas (i.e., CpG islands), which are frequently located in promoter regions. Mechanisms by which DNA methylation regulates gene transcription and cellular function are complex, and exact details remain ill defined. However, as a basic principle, hypermethylation of CpG islands within promoter regions has been demonstrated to be associated with silencing of the associated gene, whilst hypomethylation favors gene expression. More specifically, at least in part DNA methylation is thought to mediate its effects via changes in the binding of transcription factors as well as its impact on the chromatin structure [4]. The main regulators of DNA methylation in mammalian cells are DNA methyltransferases (DNMTs). DNMT1 is thought to be primarily responsible for the maintenance of DNA methylation while DNMT3A and DNMT3B are considered as regulators of de novo DNA methylation [5]. A second group of enzymes involved in regulating DNA methylation are TET (ten-eleven translocation) enzymes, which have been shown to be implicated in the demethylation process by catalyzing the conversion from 5-methylcytosine to 5-hydroxymethylcytosine as a critical first step in the demethylation process [6].

It is important to recognize that epigenetic mechanisms are all closely interconnected, forming a complex system which regulates gene expression and cellular function.

DNA Methylation in the Intestinal Epithelium

As mentioned above, the intestinal epithelium plays a key role in regulating barrier function and immune homeostasis in the GI tract. In mammals, the development of a fully differentiated and functioning intestinal epithelium consists of a complex process which begins in utero with the formation of a pseudostratified epithelial cell layer derived from the visceral endoderm. At the time of birth, the final crypt-villus architecture and all major cell subsets (e.g., absorptive enterocytes, Paneth cells, goblet cells, and enteroendocrine cells) have been developed. However, the epithelium remains functionally immature, requiring environmental factors such as bacterial colonization and exposure to increasingly complex food antigens in order to enter the postnatal phase of functional development [7, 8]. These early-life interactions between the epithelial cells of the host and our environment are essential for the establishment of mucosal barrier functions such as the ability of the epithelium to sense microbial stimuli and mount an appropriate immune response [9]. It is, therefore, not surprising that incomplete development or acquired impairment in intestinal epithelial cell barrier functions, potentially as a result of environmental changes, has been implicated in the pathogenesis of several intestinal diseases, including necrotizing enterocolitis and IBD [9–11]. The fact that these substantial functional changes occur in the absence of changes in the underlying DNA sequence suggests that epigenetic mechanisms are likely to be at play in regulating these processes.

Indeed, evidence for this hypothesis is rapidly accumulating. A number of elegant studies in mice have demonstrated a key role of DNA methylation in regulating cellular function during intestinal epithelial development. For example, the group of Kaestner has provided major insight into the role of DNMT1, the main enzyme regulating the maintenance of DNA methylation, in the mouse intestinal epithelium. In a series of excellent studies, the group demonstrated that DNMT1 is critical for controlling small intestinal stem cell differentiation and perinatal intestinal development [12]. Loss of DNMT1 in mouse intervillus progenitor cells was found to cause global hypomethylation, premature differentiation, and apoptosis, ultimately leading to loss of nascent villi [13].

Constant exposure as well as direct cross talk between the intestinal epithelium and the gut microbiota has long been suggested to drive epigenetic programming of the host epithelial cell. Indeed, recent work by Yu et al. [14] provided direct evidence for this plausible concept. Specifically, the group not only confirmed a critical role for DNMT1 in regulating mouse intestinal epithelial stem cell function but also demonstrated that exposure to the gut microbiome during the suckling period was critical for epigenetic programming and functional development. Further evidence for the important role of the gut microbiota in modulating the intestinal epithelial epigenome was provided by

Takahashi et al. [15], who were able to show that low responsiveness of human intestinal epithelial cells to lipopolysaccharides was mediated by downregulation of toll-like receptor (TLR4) gene transcription through epigenetic mechanisms, in this case histone deacetylation and DNA methylation. Moreover, using a germ-free mouse model, the authors went on to demonstrate that epigenetic regulation of TLR4 in colonic intestinal epithelial cells was at least in part controlled by commensal bacteria [16]. Together these studies clearly highlight how microbial-epithelial cross talk regulates intestinal epithelial cellular function mediated via epigenetic mechanisms.

Compared to data generated using animal models, relatively little information is currently available on human tissue/cells. This may be due to the major challenge of separating out sufficient numbers of a specific cell type of interest from mixed cell tissue samples. Given that epigenetic signatures are highly cell type specific, significant changes in the cellular composition within a mixed cell sample represent a major confounding factor. Purification of individual cell types is, therefore, highly desirable, not only to avoid detecting a signal caused by changes in cellular composition (e.g., comparing inflamed versus noninflamed tissue samples) but also to allow cell type-specific epigenetic changes to be detected.

In order to address this issue, we established a suitable protocol for the purification of intestinal epithelium from mucosal biopsies, allowing us to perform DNA methylation analysis in primary purified human intestinal epithelium [17]. By comparing methylation profiles of human fetal and pediatric intestinal epithelium using this protocol, we went on to demonstrate that DNA methylation plays a major role in regulating gene expression and cellular function in the intestinal epithelium during physiological GI development [18]. The generated genome-wide DNA methylation signatures allowed us to identify a large number of differentially methylated regions which also displayed significant changes in their gene expression. Interestingly, many of these regulatory differentially methylated regions were found within genes known to be involved in intestinal epithelial innate defense, e.g., TLR3, polymeric immunoglobulin receptor, and mucin 2 (MUC2). Moreover, performing pathway analysis on regulatory differentially methylated regions revealed a significant enrichment of genes associated with GI and immunological diseases, suggesting that alterations in the epigenetic (i.e., DNA methylation) programming during physiological GI development could lead to the development of disease in later life. Indeed, a developmental origin is increasingly being implicated in the pathogenesis of many multifactorial, complex diseases including IBD. Our findings suggest that this might at least in part be mediated by epigenetic mechanisms (Fig. 1).

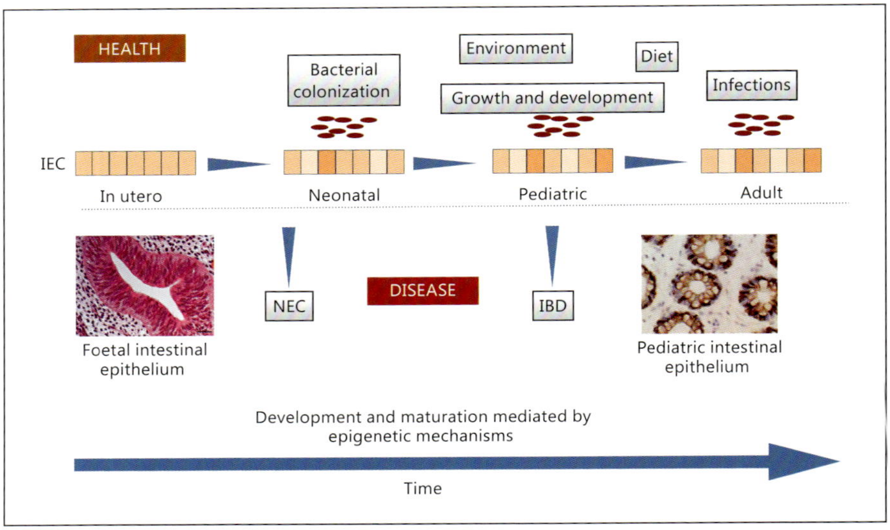

Fig. 1. Role of epigenetic mechanisms during intestinal epithelial development. The human intestinal epithelium undergoes both morphological and molecular changes during physiological development. Exposure to various environmental factors is essential during this process and has been shown to modulate epigenetic programming. Alterations may lead to the development of associated disease such as inflammatory bowel disease (IBD) and necrotizing enterocolitis (NEC). IEC, intestinal epithelial cells.

Epigenetics in Inflammatory Bowel Disease

IBD causes chronic gut inflammation of the large bowel (ulcerative colitis) or the entire intestinal tract (Crohn disease). Over the last decades, there has been a significant increase in the incidence of IBD not only in the Western world, but also in developing countries and particularly in those adapting to a more Western lifestyle [19]. Moreover, this increase is particularly alarming in patients diagnosed during childhood, given that many of these present with a much more severe phenotype [20, 21]. Genome-wide association studies have successfully linked over 160 genetic susceptibility loci to IBD [22]. However, the vast majority of these loci contributes to disease development with low odds ratios (1–1.5), suggesting a limited genetic attribution to these disorders. Moreover, observations in monozygotic twins revealed a low concordance of <50% for IBD within pairs [23]. Together, these facts highlight that environmental factors are likely to play an important role in the development of IBD and, combined with a stable human genome, directly implicate epigenetic mechanisms in disease pathogenesis [24].

Despite the plausible concept, current evidence remains limited to a small number of studies reporting changes in the DNA methylation profile in the inflamed/affected versus noninflamed intestinal mucosa of IBD patients and healthy controls [25, 26]. While these reports provide further support of epigenetics playing an important role in disease pathogenesis, the fact that all of these studies were performed on mixed cell tissue samples does not allow the identification of specific cell types, which might harbor alterations in their epigenetic profiles.

Over the last 4 years, we have recruited a large cohort of children newly diagnosed with IBD as well as matched controls. Using our established method of purifying the intestinal epithelium from intestinal forceps biopsies, we performed genome-wide methylation profiling on epithelial cell samples obtained from gut segments which are frequently affected by IBD (i.e., terminal ileum and sigmoid colon). Interestingly, unsupervised clustering analysis of genome-wide DNA methylation profiles revealed a clear separation of patient-derived colonic epithelial samples in two distinct subgroups: one group clustering together with all samples obtained from healthy children, while the second group consists exclusively of intestinal epithelium obtained from children newly diagnosed with IBD. Importantly, the observed clustering pattern did not entirely depend on the presence or absence of inflammation [18].

Following up on our findings from human fetal and healthy pediatric epithelium, we aimed to test the hypothesis that altered epigenetic programming could be implicated in IBD pathogenesis. Indeed, we observed a highly significant overlap between genes undergoing dynamic DNA methylation changes during physiological intestinal epithelial development (i.e., during the transition from human fetal to healthy pediatric epithelium) with those genes displaying altered epigenetic profiles in children diagnosed with IBD.

As part of our current work, we are further investigating the biological as well as clinical relevance of the observed DNA methylation changes in a subset of children diagnosed with IBD. We speculate that intestinal epithelial DNA methylation profiles may reflect distinct phenotypic subgroups of patients and hence might be helpful as disease prognostic biomarkers in predicting disease outcome.

Human Intestinal Epithelial Organoids

Despite the major insight gained by analysis of primary human tissue, investigating specific functional mechanisms requires the use of appropriate in vivo and/or in vitro model systems.

Recent ground-breaking discoveries in the field of stem cell biology have led to the development of novel, three-dimensional organoid culture models. Among those are intestinal epithelial organoids, which can be derived from either adult stem cells (i.e., located in the intestinal mucosal crypt

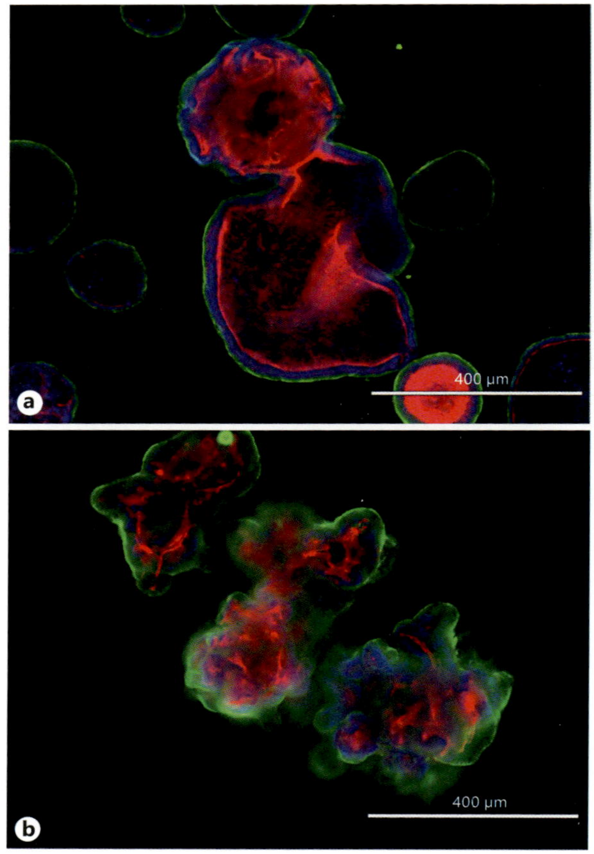

Fig. 2. Human intestinal epithelial organoids. Self-organizing, three-dimensional organoids derived from fetal distal gut (**a**) and pediatric ileum (**b**) stained for the epithelial cell adhesion molecule Ep-CAM (green), actin filament (red) and cellular nuclei (blue). Scale bar, 400 µm.

compartment) or pluripotent stem cells (i.e., embryonic or induced pluripotent stem cells). The possibility to generate such organoids from patients diagnosed with related GI diseases opens up unprecedented opportunities to investigate intestinal epithelial cell (patho)biology. Moreover, combining organoid culture systems with recently developed genome-editing tools (e.g., CRISPR/Cas9) provides an ideal platform to perform functional analysis in a human cell system.

Over the last 2 years and in close collaboration with some of the leaders in the field of stem cell biology (i.e. Dr. B.K. Koo and Prof. L. Vallier, Cambridge Stem Cell Institute), we have established a human intestinal epithelial organoid culture system in our group. We are now able to generate intestinal epithelial organoid cultures from mucosal biopsies derived from different gut segments as well as human fetal gut samples (Fig. 2). Additionally, we have started to generate a biobank of organoid cultures derived from healthy individuals as well as patients newly diagnosed with IBD, providing us with exciting novel opportunities to perform translational research in the epigenetics of IBD and potentially other related conditions.

Summary and Future Perspective

Epigenetic mechanisms are increasingly being recognized as operating at the interface between our environment and the human genome. Their crucial role in orchestrating GI homeostasis and driving physiological development, as well as underlying potential disease pathogenesis is becoming ever more apparent. Despite the major challenges still facing researchers and clinicians performing translational, epigenetic research, we are at the start of a new era where novel techniques and insights will further advance our understanding of human biology and disease.

Disclosure Statement

The authors declare no conflict of interest.

References

1 Waddington CH: Canalization of development and the inheritance of acquired characters. Nature 1942;150:563–565.
2 Heard E, Martienssen RA: Transgenerational epigenetic inheritance: myths and mechanisms. Cell 2014;157:95–109.
3 Tessarz P, Kouzarides T: Histone core modifications regulating nucleosome structure and dynamics. Nat Rev Mol Cell Biol 2014;15:703–708.
4 Schübeler D: Function and information content of DNA methylation. Nature 2015;517:321–326.
5 Bird A: DNA methylation patterns and epigenetic memory. Genes Dev 2002;16:6–21.
6 Tahiliani M, Koh KP, Shen Y, et al: Conversion of 5-methylcytosine to 5-hydroxymethylcytosine in mammalian DNA by MLL partner TET1. Science 2009;324:930–935.
7 Renz H, Brandtzaeg P, Hornef M: The impact of perinatal immune development on mucosal homeostasis and chronic inflammation. Nat Rev Immunol 2012;12:9–23.
8 de Santa Barbara P, van den Brink GR, Roberts DJ: Development and differentiation of the intestinal epithelium. Cell Mol Life Sci 2003;60:1322–1332.
9 Dupaul-Chicoine J, Dagenais M, Saleh M: Crosstalk between the intestinal microbiota and the innate immune system in intestinal homeostasis and inflammatory bowel disease. Inflamm Bowel Dis 2013;19:2227–2237.
10 Cilieborg MS, Boye M, Sangild PT: Bacterial colonization and gut development in preterm neonates. Early Hum Dev 2012;88:S41–S49.
11 Salim SY, Söderholm JD: Importance of disrupted intestinal barrier in inflammatory bowel diseases. Inflamm Bowel Dis 2011;17:362–381.

12 Sheaffer KL, Kim R, Aoki R, et al: DNA methylation is required for the control of stem cell differentiation in the small intestine. Genes Dev 2014;28:652–664.
13 Elliott EN, Sheaffer KL, Schug J, et al: Dnmt1 is essential to maintain progenitors in the perinatal intestinal epithelium. Development 2015;142:2163–2172.
14 Yu D-H, Gadkari M, Zhou Q, et al: Postnatal epigenetic regulation of intestinal stem cells requires DNA methylation and is guided by the microbiome. Genome Biol 2015;16:211.
15 Takahashi K, Sugi Y, Hosono A, et al: Epigenetic regulation of TLR4 gene expression in intestinal epithelial cells for the maintenance of intestinal homeostasis. J Immunol 2009;183:6522–6529.
16 Takahashi K, Sugi Y, Nakano K, et al: Epigenetic control of the host gene by commensal bacteria in large intestinal epithelial cells. J Biol Chem 2011;286:35755–35762.
17 Jenke AC, Postberg J, Raine T, et al: DNA methylation analysis in the intestinal epithelium – effect of cell separation on gene expression and methylation profile. PLoS One 2013;8:e55636.
18 Kraiczy J, Nayak K, Ross A, et al: Assessing DNA methylation in the developing human intestinal epithelium: potential link to inflammatory bowel disease. Mucosal Immunol 2016;9:647–658.
19 Ng SC, Bernstein CN, Vatn MH, et al: Geographical variability and environmental risk factors in inflammatory bowel disease. Gut 2013;62:630–649.
20 Benchimol EI, Fortinsky KJ, Gozdyra P, et al: Epidemiology of pediatric inflammatory bowel disease: a systematic review of international trends. Inflamm Bowel Dis 2011;17: 423–439.
21 Ponder A, Long MD: A clinical review of recent findings in the epidemiology of inflammatory bowel disease. Clin Epidemiol 2013;5: 237–247.
22 Jostins L, Ripke S, Weersma RK, et al: Host-microbe interactions have shaped the genetic architecture of inflammatory bowel disease. Nature 2012;491:119–124.
23 Khor B, Gardet A, Xavier RJ: Genetics and pathogenesis of inflammatory bowel disease. Nature 2011;474:307–317.
24 Jenke AC, Zilbauer M: Epigenetics in inflammatory bowel disease. Curr Opin Gastroenterol 2012;28:577–584.
25 Cooke J, Zhang H, Greger L, et al: Mucosal genome-wide methylation changes in inflammatory bowel disease. Inflamm Bowel Dis 2012;18:2128–2137.
26 Häsler R, Feng Z, Bäckdahl L, et al: A functional methylome map of ulcerative colitis. Genome Res 2012;22:2130–2137.

Isolauri E, Sherman PM, Walker WA (eds): Intestinal Microbiome: Functional Aspects in Health and Disease. Nestlé Nutr Inst Workshop Ser, vol 88, pp 45–53, (DOI: 10.1159/000461732)
Nestec Ltd., Vevey/S. Karger AG., Basel, © 2017

Gut-Brain Axis and Behavior

Clair R. Martin · Emeran A. Mayer

G. Oppenheimer Center for Neurobiology of Stress and Resilience, Vatche and Tamar Manoukian Division of Digestive Diseases, David Geffen School of Medicine at UCLA, Los Angeles, CA, USA

Abstract

In the last 5 years, interest in the interactions among the gut microbiome, brain, and behavior has exploded. Preclinical evidence supports a role of the gut microbiome in behavioral responses associated with pain, emotion, social interactions, and food intake. Limited, but growing, clinical evidence comes primarily from associations of gut microbial composition and function to behavioral and clinical features and brain structure and function. Converging evidence suggests that the brain and the gut microbiota are in bidirectional communication. Observed dysbiotic states in depression, chronic stress, and autism may reflect altered brain signaling to the gut, while altered gut microbial signaling to the brain may play a role in reinforcing brain alterations. On the other hand, primary dysbiotic states due to Western diets may signal to the brain, altering ingestive behavior. While studies performed in patients with depression and rodent models generated by fecal microbial transfer from such patients suggest causation, evidence for an influence of acute gut microbial alterations on human behavioral and clinical parameters is lacking. Only recently has an open-label microbial transfer therapy in children with autism tentatively validated the gut microbiota as a therapeutic target. The translational potential of preclinical findings remains unclear without further clinical investigation.

Introduction

While alterations in bidirectional brain-gut microbiota interactions are believed to be involved in the pathogenesis of well-known gut disorders such as irritable bowel syndrome (IBS) and related functional gastrointestinal (GI) disorders [1], such alterations have also been suggested to play a role in the pathophysiology of several brain disorders, including disorders of mood and affect [2], autism spectrum disorders (ASD) [2], Parkinson disease (PD) [3], and chronic pain [4]. Despite the remarkable support for such associations based on behavioral studies in mouse models of these disorders, there is limited information regarding the translational relevance of these preclinical data for human diseases. Furthermore, there are considerable gaps in our understanding of the magnitude as well as the sites, pathways, and molecular mechanisms within the gut-brain axis that are responsible for these alterations, even though candidate molecules have recently been identified which may play a role in altered social behaviors [5] and in PD [6]. The intestinal microbiota and its metabolites have been shown to be involved in modulating GI functions, given their ability to affect intestinal permeability, mucosal immune function, intestinal motility and sensitivity, and release of GI hormones and neurotransmitters from enteroendocrine and enterochromafin cells [2], as well as activity in the enteric nervous system [reviewed in 7]. Additionally, preclinical evidence suggests that the microbiota and its metabolites are likely to be involved in modulating behaviors and brain processes, including stress responsiveness [reviewed in 8], emotional behavior [reviewed in 9], pain modulation [reviewed in 2], ingestive behavior [reviewed in 10], and brain biochemistry [reviewed in 11].

To date, there is limited high-quality evidence regarding alterations in microbial ecology or production of microbial-derived metabolic products in human patients with brain or brain-gut disorders. For example, there is inconclusive evidence from human studies regarding the beneficial effects of manipulating the microbiota with prebiotics and antibiotics in patients with IBS, even though meta-analyses suggest a small therapeutic effect for probiotics [reviewed in 12]. Furthermore, it is not clear whether alterations observed in the microbiota of patients with these disorders arise from primary alterations at the gut microbial interface (bottom-up effects) and/or changes in brain-gut signaling (top-down effects).

Despite the limited clinical evidence, a large and growing number of review articles have appeared in the literature [2, 3], extrapolating the preclinical findings to human diseases. However, other than a series of case reports on the development of psychotic symptoms following broad-spectrum antibiotic intake [13], there is limited clinical evidence that acute alterations in the intestinal microbiota have an effect on clinical symptoms [reviewed in 3, 7].

This article will critically review the current preclinical literature about the role of the gut microbiota in behavior, explore the current evidence in humans consistent with the preclinical findings, and identify translational research areas required to identify a role of the gut microbiota in modulating the brain and the gut-brain axis.

Preclinical Studies

A number of experimental approaches have been employed to study the modulatory effects of gut microbiota on gut-brain interactions in experimental animals, including treatment with antibiotics [14] fecal microbial transplant [14–16], germ-free (GF) animal models [17], and treatment with probiotics. Considerable progress has been made since Sudo et al. [17] first observed that mice without normal gut microbiota exhibit marked differences in adult stress responsiveness and that these differences can be partially reversed by gut colonization. Microbiota-related effects have been reported in relation to anxiety-like behavior [5, 15, 18–23], depression-like behavior [15, 16, 22, 24], nociceptive responses [4, 25], stress responsiveness [22, 23], feeding behavior, taste preferences, and metabolic consequences [26–28].

These experimental approaches do have limitations which urge caution in translating findings to humans. GF models are born in aseptic conditions, often removed from the mother by cesarean section, and transferred immediately to an isolator in which air, food, and water are sterilized. There is a range of differences in brain and gut biochemistry [19]; blood-brain barrier permeability [29], hypothalamic-pituitary-adrenal (HPA) axis responses [17]; metabolic function [26–28]; and affective [5, 18–24], social [5, 24, 30], and ingestive [26–28] behaviors between GF animals and control animals that have normal or pathogen-free flora and who were reared by normally colonized mothers [19, 20]. The observed biochemical and behavioral changes could be mediated by a lack of gut microbiota directly or indirectly though one or several of the alterations not related to the brain.

Recent evidence suggests that the intrauterine environment is not sterile [31], and one may even speculate that the maternal gut microbial metabolites originating from the maternal gut microbiome may have an influence on fetal brain development. Furthermore, as GF pups are raised by GF mothers, the absence of fecal microbes may interfere with well-characterized maternal behaviors, such as arched-back nursing and anogenital licking. These behaviors have been associated with epigenetic changes at stress-related genes [32] that regulate the development of systems within the CNS [33]. However, in one study where maternal behavior was analyzed on days 2 and 3 postpartum, no effect of the GF status on such maternal behaviors was observed [17]. Altered signaling of the cecum to the brain, secondary to the massive cecal dilation associated with this model, could alter the development of brain regions processing such input. GF mice are leaner than control animals, despite consuming more calories [29]. Metabolic changes secondary to the loss of an important source of calories (gut microbiota-generated short-chain fatty acids) for the developing organism may affect brain development and alter the activity of brain circuits involved in feeding behavior and metabolism. Finally, the recently reported alterations in the permeability of the blood-brain barrier in GF mice is likely to result in significantly altered access of gut microbial metabolites to the brain [34]. Despite the extensive remodeling of biological systems in the GF animal, the fact that some observed behaviors and brain changes could be reversed by reconstitution of pathogen-free microbiota (conventionalization) validates some of the conclusions drawn. Nevertheless, as the GF animal has no counterpart in human brain development, premature conclusions about the translational relevance of these findings to humans should be avoided. Broad-spectrum antibiotics have well-documented transient effects on the composition and diversity of fecal microbiota [14] even though the effects on mucosa-associated microbial communities are not known.

In the studies published since 2010 using different strains of mice and rats, different strains of probiotics, and different experimental paradigms [11], a range of effects of gut microbial modulation was reported on emotional behavior [5, 15, 16, 18–24], learning and memory [22, 35, 36], social interactions [24, 30], and ingestive behaviors [27].

Emotional Behavior

When viewed together, reported findings demonstrate an increase in emotional behavior associated with infection/infestation with pathogens [18–20]; a reduction in basal or induced anxiety-like behavior in animals with normal gut microbiota, following the oral administration of probiotics [21–23, 25, 28]; and both reduced [18–20] and increased [36] anxiety in rodents raised in the absence of gut microbiota. A reduction in depression-like behaviors was observed in different rodent models with normal gut microbiota following administration of a probiotic [22, 24]. Depression-like behavior in these models was induced by maternal separation [23] and experimental myocardial infarction [24].

Learning and Memory

While improvement in impaired memory function by probiotics was observed in a rodent model of diabetes [35], several studies showed a worsening with exposure to a pathogen [36], GF status [19], and administration of a probiotic [22].

Social and ASD-Like Behavior

Gut microbiota status was found to reduce social interactions in GF mice [30], and probiotics improved social interactions in a rat model after myocardial infarction [24, 30]. Gut microbiota-associated behavioral changes were reported in different ASD mouse models, including maternal immune activation where treatment with the probiotic *Bacteroides fragilis* had a beneficial effect on some of the behavioral abnormalities [5].

Ingestive Behavior
A limited number of studies suggest that gut microbial composition can influence ingestive behavior [26, 27]. Some of these effects are likely mediated by significant alterations in GF animals in intestinal taste receptors, fatty acid receptors, intestinal transport mechanisms, and changes in the release of satiety hormones.

In addition to specific behavioral domains, effects of gut microbial modulation on CNS elements with system-wide influence were reported, including the HPA axis and signaling systems.

HPA Axis Responsiveness
Increased basal or stimulated HPA axis activity (measured as blood corticosterone or ACTH levels) was reported in GF Swiss-Webster and BALB/c mice [18, 20, 36], while a probiotic-induced reduction in corticosterone levels was observed in normal mice [22]. The association between increased HPA axis responses and reduced anxiety-like behaviors observed in several of the studies performed in GF mice suggests that hypothalamic (HPA axis) and nonhypothalamic (anxiety-like behavior) components of central stress circuits may be affected differentially by the GF conditions, depending on species and mouse strain, a response pattern not seen in the majority of existing anxiety models in which these two components of the stress response are generally congruent. One may speculate that the increased HPA axis activity in GF animals represents a response of the organism to the loss of microbiota-related energy sources, but conflicting evidence does exist [reviewed in 7].

Brain Signaling Systems
Several studies have shown reduced expression of brain-derived neurotrophic factor in the brains of GF animals (primarily in hippocampus) and increased expression in infection models. Regional changes in the expression of GABA receptor A and B subunits, NMDA receptor subunits, serotonin 1A, tryptophan, and tryptophan metabolite levels have all been reported [reviewed in 7].

Clinical Studies

Ongoing recognition of the role of the gut microbiota in preclinical models of disease, especially neuropsychiatric and metabolic diseases, demands evaluation in clinical settings. While there is a significant and growing body of literature characterizing the differences between healthy controls and individuals suffering from particular diseases, these do not help to answer the question of causality better. Studies focused on ASD, major depressive disorder (MDD), and PD have made the most significant progress towards this objective.

Autism Spectrum Disorder

The wide-ranging and variable symptoms of ASD include the difficulty with social and communicative behavior, repetitive behavior, and restricted interests. Comorbidities include intellectual disability, sleep disruption, feeding difficulty, and GI symptoms. The prevalence of GI symptoms is 9–90%, and children affected by ASD are nearly 8 times more likely to have at least one GI symptom. Moreover, GI symptom severity is strongly correlated with ASD symptom severity. These symptoms are also highly correlated with anxiety and sensory overresponsivity conditions modulated by gut microbiota in preclinical models [reviewed in 37].

Gut dysbiosis is an increasingly documented symptom of ASD, but causality remains limited to intriguing, albeit untested, hypotheses. The promising results from an uncontrolled study recently published by Kang et al. [38] showed that transfer of a standardized human gut microbiota led to reductions in GI and behavioral symptoms with a concordant maintenance of gut eubiosis, which remained 8 weeks after the intervention. Subsequent, randomized, double-blind clinical trials are essential to verify the gut microbiota as an effective therapeutic target for ASD maintenance symptoms.

Major Depressive Disorder

Preclinical studies have demonstrated the capacity of microbiota to influence parameters significant to depression pathogenesis and severity, including the levels of neurotransmitters and neuromodulators serotonin [reviewed in 39], brain-derived neurotrophic factor [17, 18, 20], and γ-amino butyric acid [22], synaptogenesis and synapse maturation [19]. Furthermore, MDD-associated gut dysbiosis is corroborated by the abnormal serum immunological parameters of depressed patients. An increased toll-like receptor 4 expression and enhanced immunoglobulin-mediated immune response to lipopolysaccharides of specific commensal bacteria implicates a "leaky gut" and increased bacterial translocation [reviewed in 39]. While studies characterizing the gut microbiome of MDD versus health have yielded marginally distinct assemblage correlations, 3 different types of studies suggest causality. Depressed human-to-rodent fecal microbial transplants have induced depressive behaviors in animal models [15, 16]; pre- and probiotic administration to healthy controls has improved anxiety and mood; and finally, incidences of *Escherichia coli* subtype outbreaks in Canada and Germany led to rises in depression and anxiety-related symptoms among the affected population [reviewed in 39].

Parkinson Disease

While the clinical hallmarks of PD remain motor deficits, there are numerous nonmotor symptoms present which contribute more detrimentally to patient quality of life. These nonmotor symptoms include psychiatric disorders, sensory alterations, and gastrointestinal problems related to dysfunctional autonomic and enteric nervous system activity. The risk of PD development increases with the infrequency of bowel movement and constipation severity. Moreover, constipation is among the earliest features, appearing as early as 15.3 years before motor dysfunction [reviewed in 40]. Early GI symptoms, thus, may be prodromal, making the gut microbiota a promising source of information for diagnosis, prognosis, and, potentially, pathogenesis. To date, clinical studies of PD and gut microbiota remain limited to characterizing the assemblage differences against healthy controls. However, Sampson et al. [6] have provided the first evidence suggesting causality by demonstrating that physical impairments in a PD rodent model are enhanced by microbiota from PD but not healthy controls.

Summary and Future Perspectives

Based on currently available evidence, there is no question that there is a relationship between the composition and function of the gut microbiota and brain function. While such a relationship has clearly been established in rodent models, the strongest evidence to date to support a significant role of such interactions in adult human subjects comes from a brain imaging study in healthy individuals and from several studies in MDD and PD patients and ingestive behavior in obesity. The majority of human studies have demonstrated associations rather than causality.

Plausible explanations for the apparent discrepancy between dramatic results in rodent models and the lack of conclusive evidence for the translatability of these findings into human disease populations include the limited homology of the human and the mouse brain in terms of brain networks relevant for human brain disorders, the limitations of the gnotobiotic mouse model, and the likelihood that brain-gut microbiome interactions in the adult are fairly stable and may have been established largely during the first 3 years of life. However, during this developmental period, there are many factors which have been shown to influence the assembly of the gut microbial architecture, including the diet and stress level of the pregnant mother, the mode of delivery, breast feeding, and early adverse life events. There is a need for large-scale, longitudinal human studies in well-phenotyped populations (including pediatric populations) as well as interventions targeted at the gut microbiome (pre- and probiotics) and the brain (mind-based therapies) to establish causality between brain and gut microbial influences.

Disclosure Statement

Emeran A. Mayer serves on advisory boards for Dannon, Danone and General Mills. Clair Martin has nothing to disclose.

References

1 Mayer EA: Gut feelings: the emerging biology of gut-brain communication. Nat Rev Neurosci 2011;12:453–466.
2 Cryan JF, Dinan TG: Mind-altering microorganisms: the impact of the gut microbiota on brain and behaviour. Nat Rev Neurosci 2012;13:701–712.
3 de Vos WM, de Vos EA: Role of the intestinal microbiome in health and disease: from correlation to causation. Nutr Rev 2012;70(suppl 1):S45–S56.
4 Amaral FA, Sachs D, Costa VV, et al: Commensal microbiota is fundamental for the development of inflammatory pain. Proc Natl Acad Sci U S A 2008;105:2193–2197.
5 Hsiao EY, McBride SW, Hsien S, et al: Microbiota modulate behavioral and physiological abnormalities associated with neurodevelopmental disorders. Cell 2013;155:1451–1463.
6 Sampson TR, Debelius JW, Thron T, et al: Gut microbiota regulate motor deficits and neuroinflammation in a model of Parkinson's disease. Cell 2016;167:1469–1480.e12.
7 Mayer EA, Tillisch K, Gupta A: Gut/brain axis and the microbiota. J Clin Invest 2015;125:926–938.
8 Dinan TG, Cryan JF: Regulation of the stress response by the gut microbiota: implications for psychoneuroendocrinology. Psychoneuroendocrinology 2012;37:1369–1378.
9 Foster JA, McVey Neufeld KA: Gut-brain axis: how the microbiome influences anxiety and depression. Trends Neurosci 2013;36:305–312.
10 Alcock J, Maley CC, Aktipis CA: Is eating behavior manipulated by the gastrointestinal microbiota? Evolutionary pressures and potential mechanisms. Bioessays 2014;36:940–949.
11 Stilling RM, Dinan TG, Cryan JF: Microbial genes, brain & behaviour – epigenetic regulation of the gut-brain axis. Genes Brain Behav 2014;13:69–86.
12 Mayer EA, Savidge T, Shulman RJ: Brain-gut microbiome interactions and functional bowel disorders. Gastroenterology 2014;146:1500–1512.
13 Weis S, Karagulle D, Kornhuber J, Bayerlein K: Cotrimoxazole-induced psychosis: a case report and review of literature. Pharmacopsychiatry 2006;39:236–237.
14 Bercik P, Denou E, Collins J, et al: The intestinal microbiota affect central levels of brain-derived neurotropic factor and behavior in mice. Gastroenterology 2011;141:599–609, 609.e1–e3.
15 Kelly JR, Borre Y, O' Brien C et al: Transferring the blues: depression-associated gut microbiota induces neurobehavioural changes in the rat. J Psychiatr Res 2016;82:109–118.
16 Zheng P, Zeng B, Zhou C, et al: Gut microbiome remodeling induces depressive-like behaviors through a pathway mediated by the host's metabolism. Mol Psychiatry 2016;21:786–796.
17 Sudo N, Chida Y, Aiba Y, et al: Postnatal microbial colonization programs the hypothalamic-pituitary-adrenal system for stress response in mice. J Physiol 2004;558:263–275.

18 Clarke G, Grenham S, Scully P, et al: The microbiome-gut-brain axis during early life regulates the hippocampal serotonergic system in a sex-dependent manner. Mol Psychiatry 2013;18:666–673.
19 Diaz Heijtz R, Wang S, Anuar F, et al: Normal gut microbiota modulates brain development and behavior. Proc Natl Acad Sci U S A 2011;108:3047–3052.
20 Neufeld KM, Kang N, Bienenstock J, Foster JA: Reduced anxiety-like behavior and central neurochemical change in germ-free mice. Neurogastroenterol Motil 2011;23:55–264, e119.
21 Bercik P, Park AJ, Sinclair D, et al: The anxiolytic effect of *Bifidobacterium longum* NCC3001 involves vagal pathways for gut-brain communication. Neurogastroenterol Motil 2011;23:1132–1139.
22 Bravo JA, Forsythe P, Chew MV, et al: Ingestion of *Lactobacillus* strain regulates emotional behavior and central GABA receptor expression in a mouse via the vagus nerve. Proc Natl Acad Sci U S A 2011;108:16050–16055.
23 Desbonnet L, Garrett L, Clarke G, et al: Effects of the probiotic *Bifidobacterium infantis* in the maternal separation model of depression. Neuroscience 2010;170:1179–1188.
24 Arseneault-Breard J, Rondeau I, Gilbert K, et al: Combination of *Lactobacillus helveticus* R0052 and *Bifidobacterium longum* R0175 reduces post-myocardial infarction depression symptoms and restores intestinal permeability in a rat model. Br J Nutr 2012;107: 1793–1799.
25 Ma X, Mao YK, Wang B, et al: *Lactobacillus reuteri* ingestion prevents hyperexcitability of colonic DRG neurons induced by noxious stimuli. Am J Physiol Gastrointest Liver Physiol 2009;296:G868–G875.
26 Duca FA, Swartz TD, Sakar Y, Covasa M: Increased oral detection, but decreased intestinal signaling for fats in mice lacking gut microbiota. PLoS One 2012;7:e39748.
27 Vijay-Kumar M, Aitken JD, Carvalho FA, et al: Metabolic syndrome and altered gut microbiota in mice lacking toll-like receptor 5. Science 2010;328:228–231.
28 Tanida M, Yamano T, Maeda K, et al: Effects of intraduodenal injection of *Lactobacillus johnsonii* La1 on renal sympathetic nerve activity and blood pressure in urethane-anesthetized rats. Neurosci Lett 2005;389:109–114.
29 Braniste V, Al-Asmakh M, Kowal C, et al: The gut microbiota influences blood-brain barrier permeability in mice. Sci Transl Med 2014;6:263ra158.
30 Desbonnet L, Clarke G, Shanahan F, et al: Microbiota is essential for social development in the mouse. Mol Psychiatry 2014;19:146–148.
31 Aagaard K, Ma J, Antony KM, et al: The placenta harbors a unique microbiome. Sci Transl Med 2014;6:237ra265.
32 Fish EW, Shahrokh D, Bagot R, et al: Epigenetic programming of stress responses through variations in maternal care. Ann NY Acad Sci 2004;1036:167–180.
33 Meaney MJ: Maternal care, gene expression, and the transmission of individual differences in stress reactivity across generations. Annu Rev Neurosci 2001;24:1161–1192.
34 Bercik P, Verdu EF, Foster JA, et al: Chronic gastrointestinal inflammation induces anxiety-like behavior and alters central nervous system biochemistry in mice. Gastroenterology 2010;139:2102–2112.e1.
35 Gilbert JA, Krajmalnik-Brown R, Porazinska DL, et al: Toward effective probiotics for autism and other neurodevelopmental disorders. Cell 2013;155:1446–1448.
36 Maes M, Berk M, Goehler L, et al: Depression and sickness behavior are Janus-faced responses to shared inflammatory pathways. BMC Med 2012;10:66.
37 Vuong HE, Hsiao EY: Emerging roles for the gut microbiome in autism spectrum disorder. Biol Psychiatry 2017;81:411–423.
38 Kang DW, Adams JB, Gregory AC, et al: Microbiota transfer therapy alters gut ecosystem and improves gastrointestinal and autism symptoms: an open-label study. Microbiome 2017;5:10.
39 Kelly JR, Clarke G, Cryan JF, Dinan TG: Brain-gut-microbiota axis: challenges for translation in psychiatry. Ann Epidemiol 2016;26:366–372.
40 Fasano A, Visanji NP, Liu LWC, et al: Gastrointestinal dysfunction in Parkinson's disease. Lancet Neurol 2015;14:625–639.

Isolauri E, Sherman PM, Walker WA (eds): Intestinal Microbiome: Functional Aspects in Health and Disease. Nestlé Nutr Inst Workshop Ser, vol 88, pp 55–56, (DOI: 10.1159/000455214)
Nestec Ltd., Vevey/S. Karger AG., Basel, © 2017

Summary of Evolution of Human Microbiota

In Session I, the presenters considered the impact of intestinal colonization, beginning in the intrauterine environment and extending into infancy, on the functions involving gut-protecting metabolic activity and the impact of brain development. *Hadar Neuman and Omry Koren* presented their extensive studies of the maternal intestinal microbiome during pregnancy. Because gut microbiota is influenced by alterations in weight, hormonal stimulation, and immunologic defenses, phenomena that occur throughout pregnancy, the maternal microbiota changes drastically from the first to the third trimester. The composition of the microbiome during the third trimester when transferred to a germ-free mouse results in an overweight, metabolically disrupted phenotype. Why these changes occur in the maternal gut during pregnancy and presumably affect the offspring as a result of the gut microbiota transmitted from the mother to the newborn during their passage through the birth canal is not known. Additional studies are needed to explain the positive impact of altered gut microbiota during pregnancy on a positive colonization of the newborn intestine.

Samuli Rautava reviewed his clinical investigations of the microbial composition of intestinal colonization in newborns under various environmental circumstances (cesarean section vs. vaginal delivery, and use of perinatal antibiotics and probiotics during pregnancy and lactation) at the time of birth. This is based on the association between intestinal composition and the expression of noncommunicable diseases (type 1 diabetes, allergy, inflammatory bowel disease, and necrotizing enterocolitis) later in life. Evidence to support this association comes from epidemiological clinical studies and studies in animal models which suggest that an abnormal initial colonization (dysbiosis) is associated with specific disease states. To more precisely show cause and effect, basic studies are required to link altered microbiota to disease mechanisms. If confirmed, this may represent a new paradigm for preventing the increased incidence of noncommunicable diseases.

W. Allan Walker summarized the importance of normal gut colonization of the newborn in immune maturation and the prevention of disease development. Factors such as birth by cesarean section, antibiotic exposure, or lack of breastfeeding may result in perturbations in the balance between potential pathogens and symbionts, termed dysbiosis, in the indigenous microbiota and eventually lead to the development of immune-mediated diseases. Supporting healthy gut colonization patterns by prebiotics or probiotics during early infancy, a critical period of development, may provide a means to reduce the risk of chronic diseases.

Matthias Zilbauer and *Judith Kraiczy*'s presentation concentrated on the role of epigenetic mechanisms and particularly DNA methylation in developmental processes in the gut and the pathogenesis of inflammatory bowel disease. Particularly epigenetic mechanisms of TLR3 signaling were discussed. Finally, they described how intestinal organoids, novel experimental gut models, have been developed and may be used to investigate intestinal physiology.

In the final talk of the session, *Clair R. Martin and Emeran A. Mayer* reviewed the current state of the knowledge regarding the so-called gut-brain axis and its influence on behavior. Data from preclinical and experimental animal studies were discussed together with novel human studies using a probiotic yoghurt product to give a comprehensive view. The approach combined neurobiology and assessment of neurotransmitters and active metabolites with behavioral measures.

Session I provided a prelude to the two subsequent sessions dealing with specific clinical conditions and suggested approaches to prevent chronic diseases using intestinal microbiota and their metabolites.

W. Allan Walker

Isolauri E, Sherman PM, Walker WA (eds): Intestinal Microbiome: Functional Aspects in Health and Disease. Nestlé Nutr Inst Workshop Ser, vol 88, pp 57–65, (DOI: 10.1159/000455215)
Nestec Ltd., Vevey/S. Karger AG., Basel, © 2017

Dysbiosis in the Neonatal Period: Role of Cesarean Section

Josef Neu
Division of Neonatology, Department of Pediatrics, University of Florida, Gainesville, FL, USA

Abstract

From epidemiological studies and studies done evaluating microbiomes in infants, there is a strong signal that the infants born by elective cesarean section (C-section) develop microbiota that differs from those babies born by vaginal delivery. Epidemiological studies show increased odds ratios for the development of immunological disorders such as type 1 diabetes, celiac disease, asthma, allergic diseases as well as metabolic diseases such as obesity in babies born by C-section. These are interesting associations, and if supported by additional studies that rigorously control for confounding factors, they will have major public health implications. Such studies represent major challenges because the confounding factors are numerous. The fact that provision of vaginal bacteria to C-section-delivered babies using a mouth swab that may actually transmit these bacteria to the infant is of interest and supports the concept that this can be done to alter the infant microbiota. However, significant caution needs to be taken, and alternative approaches that are safe as well as effective need to be considered; follow-up studies showing efficacy as well as safety need to be evaluated in the long term.

Introduction

Vaginal birth has been the natural and common mode of newborn delivery until the last century, where cesarean sections (C-sections) have become increasingly common. There are many indications for C-section delivery, both maternal and fetal ones. C-sections can be further classified into planned or emergent C-sections. Emergent C-sections are typically performed when the life of the infant or the mother can potentially be saved. States of emergency can be caused by events such as the prolapse of the umbilical cord and nonreassuring fetal heart rate tracings. Planned C-section deliveries are usually performed prior to the onset of labor and may be either medically indicated or elective. Medically indicated C-sections are generally defined as situations with a significant risk of an adverse outcome for the mother or the baby if the operation is not performed at a given time [1, 2]. Medical indications can be due to situations such as untreated maternal HIV, herpes, a history of prior uterine rupture, fetal anomalies, or abnormal fetal presentation. There are also indications which are clearly not based on medical needs, and these are usually performed secondary to convenience of scheduling for the obstetrician or family.

Although the optimal C-section delivery rate is not clear, in 1985, at a meeting organized by the World Health Organization in Fortaleza, Brazil, a panel of reproductive health experts stated that "there is no justification for any region to have a rate higher than 10–15%" [3]. Despite these recommendations, C-section rates have risen dramatically in the past 2 decades, with rates approaching 50% in some countries, such as Brazil, Iran, and the Dominican Republic. Thus, it is very likely that many of these C-sections may be unnecessary and/or simply based on convenience in countries with a high rate. Although concern should be raised in regard to the effects of these high C-section rates on the mother, their effect on public health as well as the health and maturation of the individual infants should be considered, as will be discussed in this review.

With the advent of the human microbiome project in the past decade, it has become increasingly clear that early microbial colonization will have major effects on the maturing individual. Although the term "dysbiosis" is not clearly defined, it reflects deviations from the normal microbial ecology that result in detrimental health effects on the host. Therefore, early-life perturbations of the microbiota are likely to lead to metabolic, immunological, and epigenetic consequences that have major effects on the developing individual and perhaps may even affect subsequent generations.

In this review, the effects of C-section versus vaginal delivery on the subsequent development of the microbiota, and how this relates to health outcomes, will be discussed. Studies will be presented that suggest that C-section delivery may result in a "dysbiosis" that has detrimental effects on the individual in later life. Various caveats in terms of the interpretation of the results of recent studies suggesting major differences in terms of the microbiota development and associations to subsequent health and disease will be scrutinized. These include the fact that there is considerable evidence suggesting that microbiota exists prior to delivery, and that this may also play a major role in subsequent health and disease. Furthermore, there are various environmental perturbations such as maternal diet, maternal body habitats, such as body mass index, the use of antibiotics as well as various other drugs, introduction of human milk versus donor milk versus formula, early stressors, and other factors that may play a role in confounding results of epidemiological studies as well as studies of microbiota in babies who are delivered by C-section versus vaginal delivery. In this review, we will also discuss recent methods to restore vaginal microbes after C-section delivery.

Mode of Delivery and the Infant Microbiome

Until recently, the fetal-maternal unit was believed to be sterile and only to become colonized at birth through contact with the microbial community in the vaginal canal. Thus, those infants delivered by C-section would not receive this early colonization from the vagina and required other environmental exposures to begin this colonization. However, there is ample evidence that colonization of the fetal-maternal unit begins earlier than birth since microbes have been identified in the amniotic fluid, umbilical cord blood, fetal membranes, meconium, and placenta [4]. These prenatal microbial conditions are seldom mentioned in studies comparing the effects of C-section versus vaginal delivery. In addition, differences have been found in the microbiota of children born vaginally, or by elective or emergency C-section [5]. Many of these studies suffer from interstudy methodology variability such as PCR bias and other confounding factors. Nevertheless, some of the important trends found in the literature regarding microbial composition differences in vaginally versus C-section-delivered children include: (1) children born by C-section, elective C-section in particular, exhibit diminished diversity in their microbiota; (2) less health-inducing bacterial species such as lactobacilli are seen after C-section delivery; and (3) there appears to be a trend toward more pathogenic bacteria (a possible "dysbiosis") in the developing microbiome of C-section-delivered infants.

In terms of diversity, a few studies have shown evidence of persistent negative associations between C-section delivery and infant microbial diversity and richness. In a study evaluating 16S rRNA genes in 24 healthy term infants' stool, infants born by C-section had lower total microbial diversity compared to vaginally delivered infants, and these differences persisted through the first 2 years after birth [6]. Another study in Canada using high-throughput DNA sequencing in term infant fecal samples 4 months after birth found that infants born by elective C-section had lower diversity [7]. Other studies have demonstrated higher richness in vaginally delivered infants when evaluating bacteria found in oral swab samples [8].

In 2010, Dominguez-Bello et al. [9] described the microbial communities of 10 mothers and their infants, 6 of whom were delivered by C-section. Using 16S rRNA sequencing of samples, it was found that in vaginally delivered infants, stool sample microbes collected within the first 24 h after birth most resembled their own mother's vaginal microbes. Babies who were born by C-section were colonized by bacteria that most resembled skin flora. It was suggested from this work that infants delivered by C-section lack exposure found in mother's vaginal or intestinal environment. The most dominant genera of bacteria in vaginally delivered babies when compared to those delivered by C-section were *Lactobacillus, Prevotella, Atopobium,* or *Sneathia,* whereas the most dominant genera in C-section infants was *Staphylococcus,* a common skin microbe [9]. *Lactobacillus* microbial communities are found as a dominant group in healthy vaginal communities [10]. Other studies have also found that vaginally delivered infants have more lactobacilli in the gastrointestinal tract than those delivered by C-section [11]. However, not all groups have found differences in bacterial communities in C-section versus vaginally delivered infants. In a study performed in different countries in Europe analyzing 606 infants, mode of delivery had no effect on relative proportions of bifidobacteria in 6-week-old infants [12]. In this study, infants born via C-section also had less *Bacteroides* than vaginally delivered infants. This is of interest in that *Bacteroides* may play a beneficial physiological role in the neonatal intestine [13].

There are several confounding factors that need to be taken into account in such studies (Fig. 1). Our group found that the microbiota measured in meconium during the first 48 h after birth was more diverse in preterm infants delivered by C-section [14]. This begs the question of whether meconium or samples derived within the first 24 h after birth are reasonable samples to evaluate the differences between C-section versus vaginal delivery, and whether gestational age matters in terms of the developing microbiome when related to mode of delivery. These early samples theoretically would not yet reflect microbes that are passed to the infant during the voyage through the birth canal, but rather microbes attained in utero. Again, confounding factors such as whether the C-sections were done electively or emergently, whether the mothers received antenatal or immediate postnatal antibiotics, and the length of time that either breastfeeding or formula feeding was initiated after birth are all factors that have not been fully addressed in most of these studies. The fact that many mothers are not able to provide milk for their babies shortly after birth by C-section and that colonization may differ temporally in these individuals are factors that have not been taken into account in most of the previous studies.

In conclusion, there appear to be differences in the microbial communities of infants delivered by C-section when compared to infants delivered vaginally. These differences can be persistent and can be found throughout childhood. Several of the bacteria that are found in those infants in higher quantities when

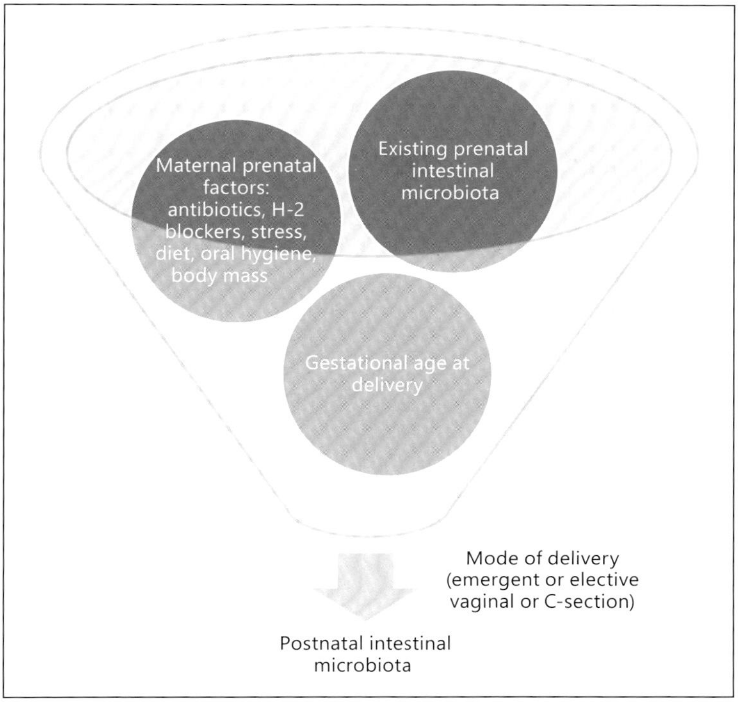

Fig. 1. Confounding factors that can affect the establishment of infant gut microbiota in addition to mode of delivery.

delivered by vaginal delivery versus C-section appear to have the known beneficial effects. However, there are confounding effects that lessen the clarity of whether the microbial differences were simply due to the process of C-section versus vaginal delivery.

Epidemiological Studies Suggesting Differences in Health Outcomes

As for short-term outcomes, there are little data to support that C-section versus vaginal delivery results in increased complications such as necrotizing enterocolitis or infections in the immediate neonatal period. C-sections are clearly associated with increased transient tachypnea of the newborn [15]. The mechanisms for this remain unclear, and hypotheses have ranged from a lack of vaginal squeeze causing more fluid to be retained in the lungs to a lower production of chloride and other channels related to lower glucocorticoid and other hormone levels in babies delivered by C-section when compared to those infants delivered vaginally [15].

Children born by C-section have an increased susceptibility to several immune-related conditions that are seen during the 1st year after birth. These include asthma [16, 17], type I diabetes [17, 18], food allergies [16], allergic rhinitis [16], and celiac disease [19]. Other studies have found long-term associations between C-sections and non-immune-related health outcomes such as increased body mass [17, 20–22], and nervous system abnormalities [23]. Thus, there is a body of epidemiological literature that demonstrates that mode of delivery is associated with long-term health outcomes in infants and children. Nevertheless, it is important to remember that these epidemiological associations do not prove causality.

The results presented here have a high potential for overinterpretation. As illustrated in Figure 1, there are several mitigating factors that are not clearly accounted for in these studies. The initial medical reason for the C-section and the socioeconomic status of the mother and family may play a significant role as to whether the infant is delivered by C-section versus vaginal delivery. Socioeconomic status and race have also been shown to play a role in the development of different microbiomes [24]. Stress and its subsequent effects on lactation [25] experienced by mothers who eventually have C-section instead of vaginal delivery are also not accounted for in these epidemiological studies. Most babies born by C-section in the United States also received a dose of antibiotics either shortly before or after delivery in order to prevent maternal infection [26]. If the mother is breastfeeding these antibiotics may get transferred through the breast milk to the infant and this may alter the microbiota of the newly born infant. Furthermore, those infants who were born by C-section may have mothers who are not able to produce breast milk for 3–5 days versus vaginally born infants whose mothers are able to produce milk usually within the first 24 h after birth [27]. Delayed breastfeeding in the C-section-delivered infants may contribute to the altered development of the microbiota, as well as very early immunological alterations that may affect subsequent health. Such confounding factors need to be accounted for in order to decrease skepticism for studies that suggest later immunological or metabolic diseases that differ because of the mode of delivery and modulation of the infant microbiome.

Strategies for Restoration of the Vaginal Microbes in C-Section-Delivered Infants

If exposure to vaginal microbes during vaginal delivery results in colonization with vaginal microbes and C-section does not, an obvious remedy would be to expose infants born by C-section to vaginal microbes. A recent pilot study sought to recapitulate infants' initial encounter with vaginal microbiota right after birth using a technique where gauze that was preincubated in the maternal vagina for 1 h and then applied to the baby's mouth, face, and body immediately after C-section birth [28]. The composition of the microbiota in infants born by C-section with and without the gauze restoration procedure was compared to vaginally born infants. The gauze treatment restored the presence of vaginal-type bacteria in C-section-delivered infants. Of interest is the fact that anal samples of C-section-delivered exposed babies were not different from unexposed babies. All newborns including those born by vaginal delivery had an abundance of bacteria categorized as gut derived when evaluated immediately after birth. It is unlikely that the meconium samples of C-section-delivered babies, as well as those from the gauze-exposed C-section-delivered babies or vaginally delivered babies, in any way represented the vaginal microbiota since this would more likely represent in utero environment rather than extrauterine environmental modification.

This study did have several limitations, one of which was the very small number of subjects with only 4 of the C-section-delivered babies exposed to the gauze microbial restoration technique. All mothers undergoing C-section had cephalosporin antibiotics administered whereas those who delivered vaginally had not. Furthermore, the decision whether or not to deliver by C-section may have been made because of specific medical indications, and this was not clearly delineated in this study. The effect of breastfeeding and length of time to establish breastfeeding in these mothers and infants was also not evaluated. Nevertheless, this study is an important first step for proof of concept that the microbial colonization of the vaginal tract can be transferred to infants who were born by C-section delivery.

Clearly, this is not a technique that is ready for routine use despite many parents already requesting this be done for their infants. Parents and physicians need to recognize inherent safety concerns with this technique. For example, even if the mother's serology is group B *Streptococcus* negative, this should not rule out the possibility of exposure because many cases where group B streptococci had led to death were in infants whose mothers' serologies were negative [29]. Undetected herpes or HIV may also be of concern. If the mother has primary herpes which is undetected, and the infant is born vaginally, the chances of death from fulminant systemic herpes infection in that infant are high.

Breastfeeding confers a set of microbes to the newborn infant. Breast milk is known to contain microbes that may play a role in infant health [30]. The study by Azad et al. [7] shows that by 4 months after birth, breastfeeding leads to a microbial colonization in C-section-delivered babies that is somewhat similar to that of vaginally delivered babies [7]. However, none of these techniques have thus far been demonstrated to provide a short- or long-term subsequent benefit.

Concluding Remarks

From this review, it is obvious that there is a strong signal that infants born by elective C-section develop microbiota that differs from those babies born by vaginal delivery. This is seen in association with epidemiological studies that show increased odds ratios of immunological and metabolic diseases in those babies born by C-section versus vaginal delivery. This may have major public health implications. However, there are major difficulties with the interpretation of these results from both the epidemiological and the microbiota-oriented studies since there are numerous confounding factors that are difficult to control. Studies that tightly control for these factors still need to be done. The fact that provision of vaginal bacteria to C-section-delivered babies using a mouth swab may actually transmit these bacteria to the infant is of interest, but caution is advised, and alternative approaches need to be developed that are safe as well as effective. Follow-up studies showing efficacy as well as safety need to be evaluated in long-term studies.

Acknowledgment

The author was supported by a Scientific Advisory Board and Research Grant from Medela, a Research Grant from Infant Bacterial Therapeutics, and by the Scientific Advisory Board of Nutricia.

Disclosure Statement

The author has no conflict of interest.

References

1 Lavender T, Hofmeyr GJ, Neilson JP, et al: Caesarean section for non-medical reasons at term. Cochrane Database Syst Rev 2012; 3:CD004660.

2 Rossignol M, Moutquin JM, Boughrassa F, et al: Preventable obstetrical interventions: how many caesarean sections can be prevented in Canada? J Obstet Gynaecol Can 2013;35:434–443.

3 Appropriate technology for birth. Lancet 1985;2:436–437.

4 Neu J: The microbiome during pregnancy and early postnatal life. Semin Fetal Neonatal Med 2016;21:373–379.

5 Stokholm J, Thorsen J, Chawes BL, et al: Cesarean section changes neonatal gut colonization. J Allergy Clin Immunol 2016;138:881–889.e2.

6 Jakobsson HE, Abrahamsson TR, Jenmalm MC, et al: Decreased gut microbiota diversity, delayed Bacteroidetes colonisation and reduced Th1 responses in infants delivered by caesarean section. Gut 2013;63:559–566.

7 Azad MB, Konya T, Maughan H, et al: Gut microbiota of healthy Canadian infants: profiles by mode of delivery and infant diet at 4 months. CMAJ 2013;185:385–394.

8 Lif Holgerson P, Harnevik L, Hernell O, et al: Mode of birth delivery affects oral microbiota in infants. J Dent Res 2011;90:1183–1188.

9 Dominguez-Bello MG, Costello EK, Contreras M, et al: Delivery mode shapes the acquisition and structure of the initial microbiota across multiple body habitats in newborns. Proc Natl Acad Sci U S A 2010;107:11971–11975.

10 DiGiulio DB, Callahan BJ, McMurdie PJ, et al: Temporal and spatial variation of the human microbiota during pregnancy. Proc Natl Acad Sci U S A 2015;112:11060–11065.

11 Pandey PK, Verma P, Kumar H, et al: Comparative analysis of fecal microflora of healthy full-term Indian infants born with different methods of delivery (vaginal vs cesarean): *Acinetobacter* sp. prevalence in vaginally born infants. J Biosci 2012;37:989–998.

12 Fallani M, Young D, Scott J, et al: Intestinal microbiota of 6-week-old infants across Europe: geographic influence beyond delivery mode, breast-feeding, and antibiotics. J Pediatr Gastroenterol Nutr 2010;51:77–84.

13 Biasucci G, Benenati B, Morelli L, et al: Cesarean delivery may affect the early biodiversity of intestinal bacteria. J Nutr 2008;138: 1796S–1800S.

14 Ardissone AN, de la Cruz DM, Davis-Richardson AG, et al: Meconium microbiome analysis identifies bacteria correlated with premature birth. PLoS One 2014;9:e90784.

15 Jain L, Eaton DC: Physiology of fetal lung fluid clearance and the effect of labor. Semin Perinatol 2006;30:34–43.

16 Cho CE, Norman M: Cesarean section and development of the immune system in the offspring. Am J Obstet Gynecol 2013;208: 249–254.

17 Hyde MJ, Mostyn A, Modi N, Kemp PR: The health implications of birth by Caesarean section. Biol Rev Camb Philos Soc 2012;87:229–243.

18 Paun A, Yau C, Danska JS: Immune recognition and response to the intestinal microbiome in type 1 diabetes. J Autoimmun 2016; 71:10–18.

19 Decker E, Engelmann G, Findeisen A, et al: Cesarean delivery is associated with celiac disease but not inflammatory bowel disease in children. Pediatrics 2010;125:e1433–e1440.

20 Goldani HA, Bettiol H, Barbieri MA, et al: Cesarean delivery is associated with an increased risk of obesity in adulthood in a Brazilian birth cohort study. Am J Clin Nutr 2011;93:1344–1347.

21 Ajslev TA, Andersen CS, Gamborg M, et al: Childhood overweight after establishment of the gut microbiota: the role of delivery mode, pre-pregnancy weight and early administration of antibiotics. Int J Obes (Lond) 2011;35: 522–529.

22 Mesquita DN, Barbieri MA, Goldani HA, et al: Cesarean section is associated with increased peripheral and central adiposity in young adulthood: cohort study. PLoS One 2013;8:e66827.

23 Kapellou O: Effect of caesarean section on brain maturation. Acta Paediatr 2011;100: 1416–1422.

24 Cassidy-Bushrow AE, Wegienka G, Havstad S, et al: Race-specific association of caesarean-section delivery with body size at age 2 years. Ethn Dis 2016;26:61–68.

25 Ahlqvist-Bjorkroth S, Vaarno J, Junttila N, et al: Initiation and exclusivity of breastfeeding: association with mothers' and fathers' prenatal and postnatal depression and marital distress. Acta Obstet Gynecol Scand 2016;95: 396–404.

26 Smaill FM, Gyte GM: Antibiotic prophylaxis versus no prophylaxis for preventing infection after cesarean section. Cochrane Database Syst Rev 2010;1:CD007482.

27 Kearney MH, Cronenwett LR, Reinhardt R: Cesarean delivery and breastfeeding outcomes. Birth 1990;17:97–103.

28 Dominguez-Bello MG, De Jesus-Laboy KM, Shen N, et al: Partial restoration of the microbiota of cesarean-born infants via vaginal microbial transfer. Nat Med 2016;22:250–253.

29 Gervasio CT, Mantaring BS, Alankar S, Shankaran S: Early-onset neonatal group B streptococcal sepsis: intrapartum antibiotic prophylaxis in the clinical setting. J Perinatol 2001;21:9–14.

30 Gomez-Gallego C, Garcia-Mantrana I, Salminen S, Collado MC: The human milk microbiome and factors influencing its composition and activity. Semin Fetal Neonatal Med 2016;21:400–405.

Isolauri E, Sherman PM, Walker WA (eds): Intestinal Microbiome: Functional Aspects in Health and Disease. Nestlé Nutr Inst Workshop Ser, vol 88, pp 67–79, (DOI: 10.1159/000455216)

Early-Life Antibiotic Exposure, Gut Microbiota Development, and Predisposition to Obesity

Meghan B. Azad[a, c] • Shirin Moossavi[b, d] • Arthur Owora[a, c, e] • Shadi Sepehri[c]

Departments of [a]Pediatrics and Child Health and [b]Medical Microbiology, University of Manitoba, and [c]Manitoba Developmental Origins of Chronic Diseases in Children Network (DEVOTION), Children's Hospital Research Institute of Manitoba, Winnipeg, MB, Canada; [d]Digestive Oncology Research Center, Digestive Disease Research Institute, Tehran University of Medical Sciences, Tehran, Iran; [e]Department of Public Health, Syracuse University, New York, NY, USA

Abstract

Antibiotics are often prescribed inappropriately to infants and young children, with potentially adverse effects on the developing gut microbiota and related metabolic processes. We review evidence from 17 epidemiologic studies suggesting that antibiotic exposure during critical periods of early development may influence weight gain and the development of obesity. Complementary research in both humans and rodents indicates that gut microbiota play a key role in this process, although further research is needed to confirm and characterize the causal mechanisms involved. Obesity is a complex and multifactorial condition; thus, a multipronged prevention strategy will be required to curb the current obesity epidemic. Evidence to date suggests this strategy should include the judicious use of antibiotics, especially in early life when the developing gut microbiota is particularly susceptible to perturbations with long-lasting implications for metabolic programming and obesity risk.

Introduction

Obesity is a major public health challenge in both developed and developing countries. Global obesity prevalence is expected to reach 20% by 2025 [1], placing over 1 billion individuals at risk for obesity-related complications, including cardiovascular disease and diabetes. Accumulating evidence indicates that

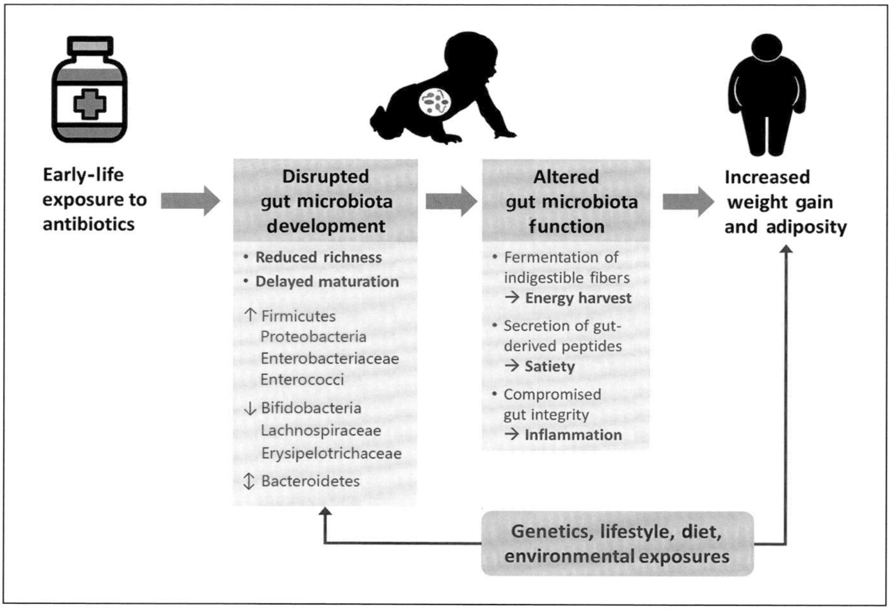

Fig. 1. Early-life antibiotic exposure, gut microbiota, and development of obesity. Schematic summary of observed associations in human and rodent studies.

weight gain trajectories are "programmed" in early life, and that gut microbiota play a key role in this process [2–5]. Antibiotics could therefore impact weight gain and obesity risk by disrupting the normal colonization and development of gut microbiota during critical phases of prenatal and postnatal development. Here, we summarize the evidence for this hypothesis from recent epidemiologic and clinical studies, as well as experimental research in rodent models (Fig. 1).

Epidemiologic Evidence: Early-Life Antibiotics and Subsequent Obesity

Antibiotics have been used as growth promoters in the farming industry for decades [6], but this phenomenon had not been studied in humans until 2011 when Ajslev et al. [7] reported an increased risk of overweight among school-age children who had received antibiotics during infancy. Several subsequent studies in different settings have provided further evidence of this association (Table 1).

Three population-based prospective cohort studies in the UK [8], Denmark [7], and The Netherlands [9] have found that antibiotic exposure during the first 6 months of life is significantly associated with increased weight gain,

Table 1. Summary of epidemiologic studies evaluating early-life antibiotic exposure and anthropometric outcomes

Study, year	Setting	*n*	Timing of antibiotic exposure	Anthropometric outcome	Age at outcome assessment	Main finding
Ajslev et al. [7], 2011	Denmark	28,354	<6 months	Overweight, obesity	7 years	Increased risk of overweight, only in children of normal-weight mothers
Trasande et al. [8], 2013	UK	11,532	<24 months	BMI, overweight, obesity	0–7 years	Increased BMI and risk of overweight with exposure before 6 months
Bailey et al. [12], 2014	USA	64,580	<24 months	BMI, obesity	2–5 years	Increased risk of obesity; cumulative effects; stronger effects with earlier exposures
Azad et al. [17], 2014	Canada	616	<12 months	Overweight, central adiposity	12 years	Increased risk of overweight and high central adiposity, only in boys
Murphy et al. [18], 2014	18 countries	74,946	<12 months	BMI	5–8 years	Increased BMI, only in boys
Mor et al. [19], 2015	Denmark	9,886	In utero	Overweight, obesity	7–16 years	Increased risk of overweight and obesity; stronger effects in boys; differences according to birth weight
Mueller et al. [20], 2015	USA	436	In utero	BMI, obesity, adiposity	7 years	Increased BMI, adiposity, and risk of obesity
Krenz-Niedbala et al. [21], 2015	Poland	1,277	<12 months	Obesity	8 years	Increased risk of obesity
Saari et al. [13], 2015	Finland	12,062	<24 months	BMI, height, weight, overweight	0–2 years	Increased BMI; stronger effects in boys, with earlier exposures, and for macrolides
Gerber et al. [11], 2016	USA	38,614	<6 months	Weight gain	0–8 years	No association
Mbakwa et al. [9], 2016	The Netherlands	979	<10 years	Height, weight, BMI, overweight	0–10 years	Increased weight and height with exposure before 24 months; no association with BMI or overweight
Scott et al. [14], 2016	UK	21,714	<24 months	Obesity	4 years	Increased risk of obesity; cumulative effects
Schwartz et al. [10], 2016	USA	163,820	3–18 years	BMI trajectories	3–18 years	Increased weight gain; reversible, persistent and progressive effects
Li et al. [16] 2017]	USA	260,556	<12 months	Obesity	1–18 years	Infections, not antibiotics, associated with obesity

Table 1. Continued

Study, year	Setting	*n*	Timing of antibiotic exposure	Anthropometric outcome	Age at outcome assessment	Main finding
Edmonson et al. [22] 2017	USA	428	2 months to 7 years	Weight, overweight, obesity	2–7 years	No association. (population 92% female)
Poulsen et al. [15] 2017	USA	8,793	In utero and <36 months	BMI	3 years	Increased BMI with postnatal exposure; cumulative effects; strongest with macrolides; no association with prenatal exposure
Ville et al. [23] 2017	USA	97	<6 months	Obesity	2 years	Increased risk of obesity

BMI, body mass index. Studies are listed in order of publication date.

overweight, or obesity later in childhood. Exposure later in infancy (after 6 months) was not consistently associated with weight gain in these studies [8, 9]. However, a recent longitudinal analysis of over 160,000 US children [10] demonstrated cumulative and persistent effects of antibiotic use on body mass index (BMI) trajectories from 3 to 15 years of age, suggesting that antibiotic use beyond infancy may continue to influence weight gain throughout childhood.

In contrast to the studies above, a registry-based US cohort study by Gerber et al. [11] found that antibiotic exposures during infancy (first 6 months) were not significantly associated with weight gain trajectories through 8 years of age. However, other registry-based studies [10, 12–15] have shown results supporting modest effects of early-life antibiotic exposure on weight gain and obesity risk. Some of these studies have also demonstrated dose-response gradients, with stronger associations from multiple exposures [12, 14, 15] and broad-spectrum antibiotics [12–15]. Most recently, findings from a large registry-based cohort study suggest that early-life infections, rather than antibiotics, are associated with an increased risk of subsequent obesity [16]. Given the limitations of administrative data sources used for registry-based studies, the observed associations are likely biased by inadequate control for confounders (such as breastfeeding, diet, and physical activity) and potential misclassification of weight-related outcomes or antibiotic exposures. However, these limitations likely bias the associations towards the null, as evidenced by the larger effect sizes reported in studies where some of these limitations were addressed [17, 18]. Notably, most of these epidemiologic studies did not distinguish between lean mass and fat mass, which is an important limitation since animal studies suggest that antibiotics may induce increased adiposity even without a change in overall body weight (see Experimental Evidence: Antibiotics, Microbiota, and Obesity in Animal Models).

New evidence suggests that in utero exposure to antibiotics may also influence weight gain. In a study of nearly 10,000 Danish school children, Mor et al. [19] reported an increased prevalence of obesity among those with prenatal exposure to antibiotics. Consistent with these findings, Mueller et al. [20] found that antibiotic exposure during gestation was associated with an increased risk of obesity at 7 years of age, along with higher BMI, waist circumference, and percent body fat. However, Poulsen et al. [15] found no association between prenatal antibiotic exposure and infant BMI at 3 years of age.

There is some evidence that antibiotic effects may be modified by infant sex or maternal BMI. Several studies have reported stronger associations in males [13, 17–19], although others found no sex differences [9, 15]. One study found that antibiotics were associated with increased obesity risk among children of normal weight mothers, while a protective association was observed among children of overweight mothers [7]. The mechanisms underlying these apparent interactions remain unexplained but may involve gut microbiota since both sex and maternal obesity are known to influence the establishment of the infant microbiota [5].

Adding to the growing body of observational evidence, Edmonson and Eickhoff [22] recently analyzed data from a randomized, placebo-controlled trial of prolonged antibiotic prophylaxis among young children at risk for recurrent urinary tract infections. In this secondary analysis, 24 months of daily trimethoprim-sulfamethoxazole treatment had no effect on weight gain or obesity. However, a single (nonmacrolide) antibiotic was tested, the median age at enrolment was 12 months, and 92% of participants were female. These factors might explain the lack of association, since observational studies have shown stronger associations from macrolides, early exposure (before 6 months), and among male infants (Table 1).

Despite the epidemiologic evidence that early-life antibiotic exposure may be associated with increased weight gain, adiposity, and obesity risk, the effect sizes are modest and the underlying mechanisms remain poorly understood. However, the hypothesized role of microbiota is supported by evidence linking gut microbiota with metabolic dysfunction, weight gain, and obesity (see Infant Gut Microbiota and Obesity), and by studies demonstrating that early antibiotic exposure can significantly and permanently alter gut microbiota profiles (see Antibiotics and the Developing Gut Microbiota). Experiments in animal models provide further supporting evidence and afford opportunities to study causal mechanisms (see Experimental Evidence: Antibiotics, Microbiota, and Obesity in Animal Models).

Infant Gut Microbiota and Obesity

Colonization of the gastrointestinal tract is critical for neonatal development and has a lasting impact on long-term health [3, 24]. This process likely begins in utero with prenatal inoculation of the infant microbiota via transmission of bacteria through the placenta and amniotic fluid [25]. Further transmission occurs through exposure to vaginal and gut microbiota during birth and milk microbiota during breastfeeding [3, 26, 27]. Initially, the neonatal microbiota is dominated by *Bifidobacteria* before gradually developing through a series of successions and replacements into a more complex and adult-like microbiota by 2 years of age [28].

Once established, the human gut microbiota can be viewed as a metabolic organ that contributes to host weight gain through several mechanisms. Gut microbiota ferment indigestible complex carbohydrates into short-chain fatty acids (including propionate, butyrate, and acetate) that can be readily used by the host colonocytes as an energy source [5]. Short-chain fatty acids and other microbial metabolites can also influence the secretion of gut-derived peptides, which consequently regulate gut motility, nutrient absorption, satiety, and energy homeostasis [29]. Finally, disturbance of gut microbiota can affect the integrity and function of the gut, resulting in translocation of lipopolysaccharides to the bloodstream and triggering low-grade inflammation, a condition that characterizes obesity and other metabolic disorders [29].

Firmicutes and Bacteroidetes are the two most abundant phyla in the mature gut microbiota. Multiple studies have reported a relative increase in Firmicutes and a decrease in Bacteroidetes among obese individuals [24, 30, 31]. Further, Ley et al. [31] demonstrated that the relative abundance of Firmicutes decreased and Bacteroidetes increased following weight loss in human subjects. At lower taxonomic levels, obesity has been associated with higher abundance of the Enterobacteriaceae family, *Prevotella, Clostridium, Eubacterium,* and *Roseburia* genera, and *Faecalibacterium prausnitzii*, and lower abundance of the genus *Bifidobacterium* [5, 30]. While the majority of this evidence has arisen from cross-sectional studies that cannot determine whether alterations in microbiota composition are a cause or consequence of weight gain, an increasing number of longitudinal studies are demonstrating that alterations in gut microbiota precede the development of obesity. Intriguingly, these changes can sometimes be detected as early as the first weeks or months of life among infants who gain excessive weight later in childhood [4, 32].

Emerging evidence suggests that disruption of normal gut microbiota development early in life may foster an "obesogenic" microbiota that contributes to the subsequent development of obesity [26]. Summarizing evidence from 8 studies investigating the association between maternal and infant gut microbiota and childhood obesity, Kozyrskyj et al. [5] concluded that higher proportions of *Lactobacillus* and lower proportions of *Bacteroides* within 3 months of birth predict a higher risk of becoming overweight later in childhood. In addition, a high abundance of *Bifidobacterium* spp. in early life appears to be associated with a lower risk of becoming overweight, whereas high abundance of *Bacteroides fragilis* increases the likelihood of obesity development [32]. Moreover, one of the strongest predictors of childhood obesity is maternal obesity [33], and a body of evidence suggests this may be partially explained by the vertical transfer of obesogenic microbiota from obese mothers to their offspring [5, 33].

With mounting evidence that gut microbiota contributes to weight gain and obesity, there is increasing interest in targeting or manipulating gut microbiota to prevent obesity or facilitate weight loss. Recognizing the importance of early gut colonization, several studies are testing new probiotic therapies (e.g. *Akkermansia muciniphila* and *Butyricicoccus pullicaecorum*) in clinical trials of pregnant women [4], although further investigations are needed to fully determine the clinical safety and effectiveness of this approach. Alongside these attempts to optimize gut microbiota with probiotics, there is a strong interest in understanding and mitigating the impact of antibiotics on the developing gut microbiota (see next section).

Antibiotics and the Developing Gut Microbiota

Gut colonization is influenced by perinatal and postnatal antibiotic exposure [26, 32]. Even the relatively stable and resilient adult gut microbiota can undergo persistent changes following repeated antibiotic exposures [34], but the infant gut microbiota is particularly susceptible given its transient developing state.

In many settings, intrapartum antibiotics are routinely administered as prophylaxis to women who are carriers of group B streptococci and to women delivering by cesarean section. Several small studies have demonstrated that antibiotic treatment during the intrapartum and early postnatal period can influence the developing gut microbiota. Fouhy et al. [35] reported that neonates treated with intravenous antibiotics (ampicillin and gentamicin) had higher proportions of *Proteobacterium* spp. and lower proportions of *Actinobacterium* and *Lactobacillus* spp. than untreated controls. These differences were detectable 4 weeks after treatment, and while most changes had resolved by 8 weeks, the shift in Proteobacteria persisted. Consistent with these results, Arboleya et al. [36] found that both maternal intrapartum antibiotics and neonatal antibiotic treatment were associated with an increased abundance of Enterobacteriaceae during the first 3 months of life. Maternal intrapartum antibiotics have also been associated with depletion of *Bifidobacterium* spp. and reduced bacterial richness 1 week after birth [37]. Recent results from the larger Canadian Healthy Infant Longitudinal Development (CHILD) study further demonstrate the impact of intrapartum antibiotics on infant microbiota, showing depletion of *Bacteroides* and enrichment of *Enterococcus* at 3 months of age [38].

Studies in older infants and children also show long-lasting effects of early antibiotic exposure. Bokulich et al. [28] recently profiled the gut microbiota development of 43 US infants during the first 2 years of life and found that antibiotic exposure during the first 12 months was associated with delayed microbiota maturation, characterized by the depletion of Lachnospiraceae and Erysipelotrichaceae, which in turn altered the functional capacity of the microbial community. Korpela et al. [39] examined antibiotic-induced alterations of gut microbiota in 142 Finnish children (2–7 years old) and found that macrolide use was associated with long-lasting shifts in gut microbiota, including depletion of Actinobacteria and enrichment of Bacteroidetes and Proteobacteria. Overall microbiota richness and maturity were also reduced and remained lower than in controls, even 2 years after exposure. Weaker effects and more rapid recovery were observed in the Finnish study following penicillin versus macrolide exposure, indicating that different antibiotics have distinct effects on gut microbiota. In both studies, stronger effects were observed when exposure occurred in the first 6 months of life, suggesting that a critical window exists where antibiotic exposure is particularly damaging to the developing gut microbiota.

Surprisingly little is known about the impact of in utero antibiotic exposure on the infant gut microbiota, although this is an area of growing interest given the widespread use of antibiotics during pregnancy [40], increasing knowledge of maternal-infant transfer of microbiota (see Infant Gut Microbiota and Obesity), and emerging evidence that even prenatal antibiotic exposure is associated with the risk of obesity (see Epidemiologic Evidence: Early-Life Antibiotics and Subsequent Obesity).

Experimental Evidence: Antibiotics, Microbiota, and Obesity in Animal Models

Animal models provide the opportunity to precisely control the dose and timing of antibiotic exposure, determine their impact on weight gain, and study the underlying biological mechanisms, including the role of gut microbiota. Blaser and his group have characterized the impact of early-life antibiotic exposure in a series of experiments using rodent models [41–44]. Initially, mice were given subtherapeutic antibiotic treatment (STAT) with penicillin, vancomycin, or chlortetracycline to mimic the regular practice in farm animals [41]. STAT was initiated at weaning (4 weeks of age) and did not affect total body mass; however, a significant increase in fat mass and percent body fat was observed with penicillin or chlortetracycline treatment. Fecal microbiota composition was also substantially modified by STAT, including an increase in the ratio of Firmicutes to Bacteroidetes [41].

Next, to examine the importance of the timing of antibiotic exposure, STAT was initiated either at birth or at weaning [42]. Accelerated growth, increased total body mass, and elevated abdominal and visceral adiposity were observed when mice were exposed from birth, while lesser effects were seen with later exposure. Weight gain and fat mass accumulation were further enhanced in STAT mice when a high-fat diet was introduced in adulthood. Consistent with epidemiologic findings (see Epidemiologic Evidence: Early-Life Antibiotics and Subsequent Obesity), more pronounced effects were seen in males for some outcome measures. STAT also perturbed the fecal microbiota, including relative enrichment of Bacteroidetes and Proteobacteria and depletion of Firmicutes. At the genus level, *Anaeroplasma*, *Coprobacillus*, *Oscillospira*, and *Ruminococcus* were enriched in STAT mice while *Lactobacillus*, *Prevotella*, *Allobaculum*, and *Candidatus Arthromatus* were enriched in controls. Interestingly, STAT-induced microbiota shifts generally resolved after STAT exposure was terminated, yet the metabolic phenotypes persisted. These sustained effects on body composition indicate that microbiota disruption in early life can have a long-term impact on the obesity risk, even when the microbiota appears to recover from the perturbation.

Microbiota transplant experiments were performed to demonstrate a causal role for microbiota in the obesogenic effect of early-life STAT [42], showing that germ-free mice colonized with microbiota from STAT mice gained more weight and fat mass than controls, despite never being directly exposed to antibiotics. Mechanisms for these obesogenic effects were explored in subsequent experiments, where bomb calorimetry showed that STAT did not affect eating behavior or energy harvest in mice on a high-fat diet [43]; however, STAT mice had increased insulin resistance and altered metabolic and inflammatory profiles. In addition, STAT was associated with distinct shifts in microbiota during weaning, including a bloom of Proteobacteria, not seen in controls. STAT also significantly delayed the maturation of microbiota during the first 4 weeks of life [43].

Although prolonged STAT is routine practice on animal farms, it does not accurately reflect human usage of antibiotics. To mimic patterns of pediatric antibiotic use, a mouse model of pulsed antibiotic treatment at full therapeutic dose was established using amoxicillin (a β-lactam) or tylosin (a macrolide), reflecting the 2 most commonly prescribed antibiotic classes in children [44]. Both antibiotics moderately increased lean mass compared to controls, and, in the long term, tylosin induced a 60% greater weight change, although fat mass was not significantly affected. While the first pulse of antibiotics did not affect the microbiota maturation, the second and third pulses significantly delayed maturation compared to controls. Both antibiotics reduced the richness and evenness of bacterial communities in the short term. While amoxicillin-treated mice recovered their microbiota diversity soon after the last dose and developed a mature microbiota similar to controls, an immature and less diverse microbiota persisted in tylosin-treated mice. Similar results were recently reported by Kaliannan et al. [45], where pulsed early-life treatment with azithromycin (another macrolide) followed by a Western diet challenge led to increased weight gain, adiposity, insulin resistance, and a higher Firmicutes/Bacteroidetes ratio compared to untreated controls.

Studies examining perinatal antibiotic exposure in rodent models have also shown disruption of gut microbiota. Tormo-Badia et al. [46] treated pregnant mice with a cocktail of metronidazole, neomycin, and polymyxin and observed a persistent reduction in gut microbiota diversity among offspring. Gonzalez-Perez et al. [47] administered ampicillin, streptomycin, and clindamycin during gestation and lactation, and observed a reduction in total bacterial load accompanied by enrichment of *Enterococcus* species in the gut microbiota of offspring. Both studies showed immunological changes following perinatal exposure to antibiotics, but weight-related phenotypes were not examined.

Together, these experimental results indicate that early-life antibiotic exposure can have a lasting effect on gut microbiota, host metabolism, weight gain, and adiposity. Interestingly, these effects appear to be exacerbated by a high-fat ("Western") diet later in life. Moreover, and consistent with some epidemiologic findings, these effects appear to depend on the timing, type, dose, and duration of exposure.

Conclusions and Directions for Future Research

While antibiotics provide life-saving treatment for infectious disease, they are frequently prescribed inappropriately, especially to infants and young children [48]. Mounting evidence from epidemiologic and experimental research indicates that antibiotic exposure during critical periods of early development may influence weight gain and the development of obesity. Even with the modest effect sizes reported in some studies, these exposures could have a meaningful impact at the population level given the widespread use of antibiotics.

Results from both human and animal studies suggest that gut microbiota play a key role in the apparent association of antibiotics and obesity (Fig. 1), but further research is needed to confirm and characterize the causal mechanisms involved. For example, it will be necessary to isolate the specific microbes and microbial metabolites that influence weight gain in order to identify therapeutic targets and design effective microbiota-based intervention strategies. It is also important to recognize and study the microbiota-independent effects of antibiotics [49], and to explore the potential impact of infections (i.e., the indication for antibiotic treatment) on gut microbiota and weight gain.

Obesity is clearly a complex and multifactorial condition; thus, a multi-pronged prevention strategy will be required to curb the obesity epidemic. Based on current evidence, this strategy should include the judicious use of antibiotics, especially in early life when the developing gut microbiota is particularly susceptible to perturbations with long-lasting implications for metabolic programming and obesity risk.

Disclosure Statement

The authors declare that no financial or other conflict of interest exists in relation to the contents of the chapter.

References

1 NCD Risk Factor Collaboration: Trends in adult body-mass index in 200 countries from 1975 to 2014: a pooled analysis of 1698 population-based measurement studies with 19.2 million participants. Lancet 2016;387:1377–1396.

2 Cox LM, Blaser MJ: Pathways in microbe-induced obesity. Cell Metab 2013;17:883–894.

3 Goulet O: Potential role of the intestinal microbiota in programming health and disease. Nutr Rev 2015;73(suppl 1):32–40.

4 Isolauri E, Salminen S, Rautava S: Early microbe contact and obesity risk: evidence of causality? J Pediatr Gastroenterol Nutr 2016; 63(suppl 1):S3–S5.

5 Kozyrskyj AL, Kalu R, Koleva PT, Bridgman SL: Fetal programming of overweight through the microbiome: boys are disproportionately affected. J Dev Orig Health Dis 2016;7:25–34.

6 Jukes TH, Williams WL: Nutritional effects of antibiotics. Pharmacol Rev 1953;5:381–420.

7 Ajslev TA, Andersen CS, Gamborg M, et al: Childhood overweight after establishment of the gut microbiota: the role of delivery mode, pre-pregnancy weight and early administration of antibiotics. Int J Obes (Lond) 2011;35: 522–529.

8 Trasande L, Blustein J, Liu M, et al: Infant antibiotic exposures and early-life body mass. Int J Obes (Lond) 2013;37:16–23.
9 Mbakwa CA, Scheres L, Penders J, et al: Early Life Antibiotic Exposure and Weight Development in Children. J Pediatr 2016;176:105–113.e2.
10 Schwartz BS, Pollak J, Bailey-Davis L, et al: Antibiotic use and childhood body mass index trajectory. Int J Obes (Lond) 2016;40:615–621.
11 Gerber JS, Bryan M, Ross RK, et al: Antibiotic exposure during the first 6 months of life and weight gain during childhood. JAMA 2016;315:1258–1265.
12 Bailey LC, Forrest CB, Zhang P, et al: Association of antibiotics in infancy with early childhood obesity. JAMA Pediatr 2014;168:1063–1069.
13 Saari A, Virta LJ, Sankilampi U, et al: Antibiotic exposure in infancy and risk of being overweight in the first 24 months of life. Pediatrics 2015;135:617–626.
14 Scott FI, Horton DB, Mamtani R, et al: Administration of antibiotics to children before age 2 years increases risk for childhood obesity. Gastroenterology 2016;151:120–129.e5.
15 Poulsen MN, Pollak J, Bailey-Davis L, et al: Associations of prenatal and childhood antibiotic use with child body mass index at age 3 years. Obesity (Silver Spring) 2017;25:438–444.
16 Li DK, Chen H, Ferber J, Odouli R: Infection and antibiotic use in infancy and risk of childhood obesity: a longitudinal birth cohort study. Lancet Diabetes Endocrinol 2017;5:18–25.
17 Azad MB, Bridgman SL, Becker AB, Kozyrskyj AL: Infant antibiotic exposure and the development of childhood overweight and central adiposity. Int J Obes (Lond) 2014;38:1290–1298.
18 Murphy R, Stewart AW, Braithwaite I, et al: Antibiotic treatment during infancy and increased body mass index in boys: an international cross-sectional study. Int J Obes (Lond) 2014;38:1115–1119.
19 Mor A, Antonsen S, Kahlert J, et al: Prenatal exposure to systemic antibacterials and overweight and obesity in Danish schoolchildren: a prevalence study. Int J Obes (Lond) 2015;39:1450–1455.
20 Mueller NT, Whyatt R, Hoepner L, et al: Prenatal exposure to antibiotics, cesarean section and risk of childhood obesity. Int J Obes (Lond) 2015;39:665–670.
21 Krenz-Niedbala M, Koscinski K, Puch EA, et al: Is the relationship between breastfeeding and childhood risk of asthma and obesity mediated by infant antibiotic treatment? Breastfeed Med 2015;10:326–333.
22 Edmonson MB, Eickhoff JC: Weight gain and obesity in infants and young children exposed to prolonged antibiotic prophylaxis. JAMA Pediatr 2017;171:150–156.
23 Ville AP, Heyman MB, Medrano R, Wojcicki JM: Early antibiotic exposure and risk of childhood obesity in Latinos. Child Obes 2017, DOI: 10.1089/chi.2016.0235.
24 Garcia-Mantrana I, Collado MC: Obesity and overweight: impact on maternal and milk microbiome and their role for infant health and nutrition. Mol Nutr Food Res 2016;60:1865–1875.
25 Collado MC, Rautava S, Aakko J, et al: Human gut colonisation may be initiated in utero by distinct microbial communities in the placenta and amniotic fluid. Sci Rep 2016;6:23129.
26 Lemas DJ, Yee S, Cacho N, et al: Exploring the contribution of maternal antibiotics and breastfeeding to development of the infant microbiome and pediatric obesity. Semin Fetal Neonatal Med 2016;21:406–409.
27 Azad MB, Konya T, Maughan H, et al: Gut microbiota of healthy Canadian infants: profiles by mode of delivery and infant diet at 4 months. CMAJ 2013;185:385–394.
28 Bokulich NA, Chung J, Battaglia T, et al: Antibiotics, birth mode, and diet shape microbiome maturation during early life. Sci Transl Med 2016;8:343ra82.
29 Paolella G, Vajro P: Childhood obesity, breastfeeding, intestinal microbiota, and early exposure to antibiotics: what is the link? JAMA Pediatr 2016;170:735–737.
30 Angelakis E, Armougom F, Million M, Raoult D: The relationship between gut microbiota and weight gain in humans. Future Microbiol 2012;7:91–109.
31 Ley RE, Turnbaugh PJ, Klein S, Gordon JI: Microbial ecology: human gut microbes associated with obesity. Nature 2006;444:1022–1023.

32 Turta O, Rautava S: Antibiotics, obesity and the link to microbes – what are we doing to our children? BMC Med 2016;14:57.
33 Gohir W, Ratcliffe EM, Sloboda DM: Of the bugs that shape us: maternal obesity, the gut microbiome, and long-term disease risk. Pediatr Res 2015;77:196–204.
34 Dethlefsen L, Relman DA: Incomplete recovery and individualized responses of the human distal gut microbiota to repeated antibiotic perturbation. Proc Natl Acad Sci U S A 2011;108(suppl 1):4554–4561.
35 Fouhy F, Guinane CM, Hussey S, et al: High-throughput sequencing reveals the incomplete, short-term recovery of infant gut microbiota following parenteral antibiotic treatment with ampicillin and gentamicin. Antimicrob Agents Chemother 2012;56: 5811–5820.
36 Arboleya S, Sanchez B, Milani C, et al: Intestinal microbiota development in preterm neonates and effect of perinatal antibiotics. J Pediatr 2015;166:538–544.
37 Aloisio I, Quagliariello A, De Fanti S, et al: Evaluation of the effects of intrapartum antibiotic prophylaxis on newborn intestinal microbiota using a sequencing approach targeted to multi hypervariable 16S rDNA regions. Appl Microbiol Biotechnol 2016;100:5537–5546.
38 Azad MB, Konya T, Persaud RR, et al: Impact of maternal intrapartum antibiotics, method of birth and breastfeeding on gut microbiota during the first year of life: a prospective cohort study. BJOG 2016;123:983–993.
39 Korpela K, Salonen A, Virta LJ, et al: Intestinal microbiome is related to lifetime antibiotic use in Finnish pre-school children. Nat Commun 2016;7:10410.
40 Kuperman AA, Koren O: Antibiotic use during pregnancy: how bad is it? BMC Med 2016;14:91.
41 Cho I, Yamanishi S, Cox L, et al: Antibiotics in early life alter the murine colonic microbiome and adiposity. Nature 2012;488:621–626.
42 Cox LM, Yamanishi S, Sohn J, et al: Altering the intestinal microbiota during a critical developmental window has lasting metabolic consequences. Cell 2014;158:705–721.
43 Mahana D, Trent CM, Kurtz ZD, et al: Antibiotic perturbation of the murine gut microbiome enhances the adiposity, insulin resistance, and liver disease associated with high-fat diet. Genome Med 2016;8:48.
44 Nobel YR, Cox LM, Kirigin FF, et al: Metabolic and metagenomic outcomes from early-life pulsed antibiotic treatment. Nat Commun 2015;6:7486.
45 Kaliannan K, Wang B, Li XY, et al: Omega-3 fatty acids prevent early-life antibiotic exposure-induced gut microbiota dysbiosis and later-life obesity. Int J Obes (Lond) 2016;40: 1039–1042.
46 Tormo-Badia N, Hakansson A, Vasudevan K, et al: Antibiotic treatment of pregnant non-obese diabetic mice leads to altered gut microbiota and intestinal immunological changes in the offspring. Scand J Immunol 2014;80: 250–260.
47 Gonzalez-Perez G, Hicks AL, Tekieli TM, et al: Maternal antibiotic treatment impacts development of the neonatal intestinal microbiome and antiviral immunity. J Immunol 2016;196:3768–3779.
48 Principi N, Esposito S: Antimicrobial stewardship in paediatrics. BMC Infect Dis 2016; 16:424.
49 Morgun A, Dzutsev A, Dong X, et al: Uncovering effects of antibiotics on the host and microbiota using transkingdom gene networks. Gut 2015;64:1732–1743.

Isolauri E, Sherman PM, Walker WA (eds): Intestinal Microbiome: Functional Aspects in Health and Disease. Nestlé Nutr Inst Workshop Ser, vol 88, pp 81–94, (DOI: 10.1159/000455989)
Nestec Ltd., Vevey/S. Karger AG., Basel, © 2017

Microbiota and Necrotizing Enterocolitis

Sanjay Patole

Centre for Neonatal Research and Education, University of Western Australia, and Department of Neonatal Paediatrics, King Edward Memorial Hospital for Women, Perth, WA, Australia

Abstract

Necrotizing enterocolitis (NEC) is an acquired gastrointestinal inflammatory condition with significant mortality and morbidity in preterm very low birth weight infants. The interplay between toll-like receptors, bacterial endotoxins, developmentally regulated excessive proinflammatory responses of the immature innate immune system, hypoxia, ischemia, reperfusion, free radicals, and the presence of substrates and bacterial endotoxins is thought to play an important role in the pathogenesis of NEC. The association (cause?) of various microbes (bacteria, viruses, and fungi) with NEC has intrigued researchers for many years. Availability of newer molecular methods (e.g., 16S ribosomal RNA gene-specific primers/pyrosequencing of fecal DNA) is expected to improve our understanding of the role of gut microbiota in the pathogenesis of NEC. Recent studies employing such methods to assess fecal microbiota are reviewed. Current evidence suggests that dysbiosis of the gut microbiota precedes the development of NEC in preterm infants. Further research is required to understand the significance of changes in the gut microbiome over the early postnatal period including the relative abundance of Gammaproteobacteria and the paucity of strict anaerobic bacteria that precedes NEC in preterm infants. Assessing the reproducibility of previous findings in large prospective studies with standardized methodology (e.g. sample processing, PCR primer, and DNA extraction) is important.

Introduction

Necrotizing enterocolitis (NEC) is a potentially devastating acquired condition of the gut in preterm infants. It occurs in 4–6% of preterm infants with very low birth weight (VLBW: <1,500 g) and 9–14% of infants with extremely low birth weight (ELBW: <1,000 g) [1–6]. NEC (≥stage II) is associated with significant mortality (~25%) and morbidity including recurrent late-onset sepsis, prolonged dependence on parenteral nutrition, need for surgery, survival with intestinal failure, and long-term neurodevelopmental impairment [1–3, 7–13]. The outcomes are worse in ELBW infants needing surgical intervention for NEC [5, 9, 14]. The mortality could be as high as 100% in those with extensive full-thickness necrosis of the gut [5, 9, 14]. The socioeconomic burden of ≥stage II NEC is significant considering the prolonged hospital stay and long-term consequences of the illness [1, 15]. Advances in neonatal intensive care have resulted in an increase in the absolute number of survivors of extreme prematurity who are at high risk of NEC. Primary prevention of NEC will be difficult till prevention of preterm birth becomes a reality. The poorly understood pathogenesis of NEC makes it difficult to develop a cure for the illness [16, 17].

The interplay between various factors including the developmentally regulated inflammatory response of the immature innate immune system, hypoxia, ischemia, reperfusion, free radicals, and the presence of substrates and bacterial endotoxins is currently thought to play an important role in the pathogenesis of NEC [1, 17–22]. The roles excessive proinflammatory responses of the immature innate immune system, bacterial endotoxins, toll-like receptors, and dysbiosis of the gut microbiota play have become a research priority to improve the understanding of the pathogenesis of NEC [18, 19, 23–27]. This brief review is focused on the role of gut microbiota in the pathogenesis of NEC in preterm VLBW infants.

Role of Microbiota in the Pathogenesis of Necrotizing Enterocolitis

No specific pathogen has been consistently associated with NEC despite the wide agreement that gut microbes play an important role in the pathogenesis of this condition [28]. A range of microorganisms, including bacteria, viruses, and fungal species, has been associated with NEC in preterm infants, and the same microbe species are often found in gestation-matched healthy infants [27, 29–31]. Proving a causative relationship between a specific pathogen and NEC is thus difficult even during clustered outbreaks of the condition [32, 33]. In a prospective case-control study, Peter et al. [33] studied the association between NEC and specific pathogens. Over the study period, 18 preterm infants (<36 weeks) developed ≥stage II NEC with portal venous gas; 8 needed laparotomy, and 2 died. Gestation-matched infants without NEC were controls. In the week before NEC diagnosis, potentially pathogenic bacteria were identified in stools of all cases and 79% of controls ($p < 0.05$). There was no significant difference in the occurrence of specific pathogens or groups of pathogens in cases versus controls [33]. In the context of association versus causation, it is important to note that randomized trials of oral antibiotics to prevent NEC suggest a causal relationship between gut bacteria and NEC, and, importantly, NEC does not occur in the sterile in utero environment [34–36].

The concept of "opportunistic pathogens" suggests that a microbe that is nonpathogenic/nonvirulent in healthy term infants can become pathogenic in an immunocompromised preterm infant [37]. Leach et al. [37] investigated this issue by analyzing the meconium and fecal samples collected over the first month of life in preterm infants (24–32 weeks of gestation) by the 16S ribosomal RNA (rRNA) gene sequencing method. During the study period, 4 infants developed NEC (cases) and 18 without NEC served as controls. Fecal S100A12 concentrations, measured by immunoassay, increased significantly after NEC development. The fecal microbiome did not significantly differ in cases versus controls. However, potentially pathogenic bacteria were detected significantly more often in cases than controls ($p = 0.0007$), suggesting that they may contribute to the pathogenesis of NEC [37]. Investigators have reported that *Cronobacter sakazakii*, a gram-positive endospore-forming obligate anaerobe, is an opportunistic pathogen that displays increased virulence in a compromised host and has strain-specific effects [38–42]. The role of *C. sakazakii* in neonatal NEC is supported by studies in a rat pup model of the illness [43, 44]. Its effects are dose dependent, with higher doses (10^7 CFU) causing enterocyte apoptosis and destruction of the villus tips due to induction of proinflammatory cytokine release (e.g. IL-6) and inducible nitric oxide synthase to increase nitric oxide levels [44–46].

Studies Assessing Gut Microbiota in Preterm Infants with Necrotizing Enterocolitis

There are 17 studies [47–63] on gut microbiota in preterm NEC infants: 6 studies were published in 2016 [47–52], 5 in 2015 [53–57], 2 [59, 60] in 2013, and 1 [58, 61–63] in 2014, 2012, 2011, and 2009, respectively.

(1) In 2016, *Warner et al.* [47] reported a large prospective observational study comparing the gut bacteria in preterm VLBW infants who developed ≥stage II NEC (cases) versus those who did not (controls). The controls (1–4 per case) were matched for gestation, birth weight, and date. The primary (122 infants/2,492 stool samples) and secondary (44 infants/1,094 stool samples) cohorts were enrolled in different hospitals. They used bacterial 16S rRNA gene-specific primers and pyrosequencing of fecal DNA. A total of 28/122 infants in the primary cohort developed NEC (cases); 94 infants served as controls. The

fecal microbiota differed significantly between cases and controls after the first month of age. Development of NEC was positively associated with Gammaproteobacteria and negatively with strictly anaerobic bacteria, especially Negativicutes. In the secondary cohort, a total of 18/44 infants developed NEC (cases), and 26 infants served as controls. Combined data from all cohorts (166 infants/3,586 stools/46 NEC cases) showed increased proportions of Gammaproteobacteria ($p = 0.0011$) and lower proportions of Negativicutes ($p = 0.0013$) and the Clostridia-Negativicutes combination ($p = 0.0051$) in cases versus controls. These associations were strongest in the primary and overall cohort for infants born <27 weeks of gestation [47].

(2) In 2016, *Ward et al.* [48] reported uropathogenic *Escherichia coli* (UPEC) colonization as a risk factor for NEC and subsequent mortality. The early gut microbiota of preterm ($n = 144$) and term ($n = 22$) infants was studied using deep shotgun metagenomic sequence analysis. A pan-genomic approach was used to functionally subtype the *E. coli* and identify genes associated with NEC and mortality that indicate colonization by UPEC. Metagenomic multilocus sequence typing analysis defined NEC-associated strains as sequence types often associated with urinary tract infections, including ST69, ST73, ST95, ST127, ST131, and ST144 [48]. Further studies are needed to confirm whether there is a causal link between UPEC and NEC.

(3) In 2016, *Heida et al.* [49] studied the prognostic factors for NEC development in high-risk neonates who did (11 cases) versus those who did not (22 controls matched for gestation/birth weight) develop the illness. The 16S rRNA gene sequencing method was used. The presence and abundance of *Clostridium perfringens* (8.4%) and *Bacteroides dorei* (0.9%) in meconium were significantly increased in cases versus controls ($p < 0.001$). In postmeconium samples, the abundance of staphylococci was negatively associated with NEC; *C. perfringens* was more prevalent in NEC cases. Early enteral feeding and, in particular, breast milk were correlated with an increase in lactate-producing bacilli in postmeconium samples [49].

(4) In 2016, *Hourigan et al.* [50] reported serial microbiome changes (16S rRNA gene sequencing) in twins discordant for NEC, with similar intrauterine and early environmental exposures. A decrease in bacterial diversity and an increase in Proteobacteria were noted a week preceding the signs of NEC in the twin who developed the illness [50]. These findings suggest that early gut microbiota may play an important role in the pathogenesis of NEC.

(5) In 2016, *Cortese et al.* [51] hypothesized that a cross talk exists between the host epigenome and the initial microbiota colonizing the gut at a critical stage. By exposing immature enterocytes to probiotic and pathogenic bacteria, they showed >200 regions of differential DNA modification, which were specific

for each exposure. In a mouse model, they demonstrated that antenatal glucocorticoid treatment altered the host epigenome. The effects on the expression of genes associated with inflammatory responses and intestinal barrier function were studied by quantitative polymerase chain reaction (qPCR). The DNA modification changes in 5 candidate genes were verified by quantitative methylation-specific PCR. Using 16S RNA sequencing-based phylogenetic analysis, they showed that epigenome changes conditioned early microbiota colonization leading to differential bacterial colonization at different taxonomic levels. These findings suggest that microbial colonization may alter epigenetic signatures of the immature gut establishing inflammatory changes and compromising barrier properties predisposing to NEC [51].

(6) In 2016, *Abdulkadir et al.* [52] analyzed 72 longitudinal stool samples from 20 infants (10 NEC cases and 10 controls) by qPCR. Controls were matched for birth weight, gestation, delivery mode, and gender. There was no significant difference in the total bacterial load in cases versus controls. There were also no significant temporal changes in the total bacterial load within NEC infants before versus after NEC diagnosis, and in healthy controls [52]. These findings suggest that fecal bacterial load may not be a reliable surrogate for tissue bacterial load in NEC.

(7) In 2015, *Cassir et al.* [53] analyzed the gut microbiota in stool samples from NEC cases and controls (15 each) by 16S rRNA pyrosequencing and culture-based methods. A *Clostridium butyricum*-specific qPCR assay was developed. Stool samples from preterm infants with NEC ($n = 93$) and controls without NEC ($n = 270$) were tested. The whole genome of 16 *C. butyricum* strains was sequenced and analyzed. *C. butyricum* was specifically associated with NEC using molecular and culture-based methods (15/15 vs. 2/15; $p < 0.0001$) or qPCR (OR: 45.4; 95% CI: 26.2–78.6; $p < 0.0001$). Culture supernatants of *C. butyricum* strains from NEC infants ($n = 14$) showed significant cytotoxic activity ($p = 0.008$). A homologue of the β-hemolysin toxin gene shared by *Brachyspira hyodysenteriae*, the cause for swine dysentery, was identified in all NEC cases. The corresponding protein was secreted by a NEC-associated *C. butyricum* strain [53].

(8) In 2015, *Zhou et al.* [54] studied the longitudinal changes in the gut microbiome preceding NEC in preterm infants. Using the 16S rRNA method, they analyzed 312 samples in 12 cases that developed NEC and 26 gestation-matched controls that did not. The gut microbiome evolved rapidly during the first 2 months of life. The day of life was the major factor contributing to the colonization process. Depending on the postnatal age at development of NEC (early vs. late onset), the pattern of microbial progression was different in cases versus controls. The differences were most obvious between early-onset NEC and

controls. Closer to the onset of the illness, *Clostridium sensu stricto* was significantly more abundant in early-onset NEC than in controls. In late-onset NEC, the Gammaproteobacteria *Escherichia/Shigella* showed an increasing pattern prior to the illness and were significantly higher in cases than controls 6 days before NEC. *Cronobacter* (Gammaproteobacteria) was significantly higher in late-onset NEC cases than controls 1–3 days before NEC [54]. Overall, these results indicate that the specific pathogen associated with NEC may vary by the infant's postnatal age at onset of NEC.

(9) In 2015, *McMurtry et al.* [55] compared the gut microbiota of infants with NEC (21 cases) to matched controls without NEC (74 controls) using 454 pyrosequencing analyses of 16S rRNA genes that were PCR amplified from stool DNA specimens. NEC severity was categorized as mild, severe, and lethal. Bacterial diversity as well as the relative abundance of Actinobacteria and Clostridia was significantly lower in NEC specimens than controls. The absence of Clostridia was significantly associated with NEC. Microbial diversity and Clostridia abundance and prevalence decreased with increasing severity of NEC. The investigators concluded that low fecal bacterial diversity may be indicative of NEC and its severity, and that the presence of taxa such as Clostridia may play a role in attenuating inflammation leading to NEC [55].

(10) In 2015, *Raveh-Sadka et al.* [56] studied the spread of potential pathogens among hospitalized preterm infants in the context of NEC. They compared microbial communities between infants who did (34 cases) or did not (5 controls) develop NEC using strain-resolved comprehensive bacterial community analysis. The strains colonizing each infant were distinct, and none was common to infants who developed NEC. The investigators commented that the paucity of shared gut colonizers suggested the existence of significant barriers to the spread of bacteria among infants [56].

(11) In 2015, *Sim et al.* [57] studied the gut microbiota preceding NEC in preterm infants ($n = 369$) by next-generation sequencing of 16S rRNA gene regions. Fecal samples were analyzed from 12 infants with definite NEC, 8 with suspected NEC, and 44 controls. Before diagnosis, a clostridial operational taxonomic unit was overabundant in samples from infants with established NEC ($p = 0.006$). Culture confirmed the presence of *C. perfringens* type A. Fluorescent amplified fragment length polymorphism typing showed that no isolates were identical. Samples from NEC cases without profuse *C. perfringens* showed an overabundance of a *Klebsiella* operational taxonomic unit [57]. The utility of *Clostridium* and *Klebsiella* operational taxonomic units as biomarkers for early diagnosis of NEC needs to be confirmed.

(12) In 2014, *Brower-Sinning et al.* [58] studied the diversity of mucosal bacteria in resected gut samples from preterm infants with ($n = 16$) and without ($n =$

10) NEC, using 16S rRNA gene sequencing. The total bacterial burden was higher in NEC samples. Both NEC and non-NEC samples showed high interindividual variability and an abundance of opportunistic pathogens. The NEC samples showed an abundance of strict anaerobes and a decreased diversity of the bacterial community, and no uniform pattern of microbial colonization [58].

(13) In 2013, *Claud et al.* [59] studied the gut microbiota of preterm infants that did develop NEC (5 cases) versus those who did not (5 controls) using the 16S rRNA gene sequencing method. Over time, the gut microbiota of control infants developed and became closer to that in healthy breast milk-fed term infants. The gut microbiome differed between cases and controls, starting from 3 weeks before NEC diagnosis. The majority of the differentially abundant genes in cases were associated with carbohydrate metabolism and mapped to the Enterobacteriaceae family [59]. These findings are helpful in understanding the temporal changes in the gut microbiome and in the substrate availability for growth of different bacteria.

(14) In 2013, *Normann et al.* [60] reported no significant differences in gut microbiota composition in NEC cases versus matched controls. In a prospective study, they analyzed fecal flora by barcoded pyrosequencing in extremely preterm infants (10 cases of NEC and 20 controls matched for gender, gestation, and mode of delivery). The gut microbiota was dominated by *Enterococcus*, Bacillales, and Enterobacteriaceaea in cases, with a high relative abundance of Bacillales and Enterobacteriaceae preceding the diagnosis of NEC. The flora was dominated by enterococci in control samples. A low diversity of gut microbiota was found with no significant differences between NEC cases and controls. In 16 healthy controls, Firmicutes (*Enterococcus* and Bacillales) dominated the fecal flora during the first weeks after birth and were then succeeded by Enterobacteriaceae [60]. Further studies are needed to confirm these findings.

(15) In 2012, *Smith et al.* [61] analyzed fecal samples (n = 482) from 163 preterm infants (<30 weeks of gestation) during the first month of life by culture and PCR denaturing gradient gel electrophoresis (DGGE). A total of 21/163 infants developed NEC. Very few bacterial species could be cultured from the samples. Gram-positive bacteria dominated the samples in the NEC group, whereas in the control group a mixed flora of gram-positive and -negative bacteria were isolated. Molecular analysis using PCR-DGGE profiles did not confirm these differences. The investigators suggested that intestinal gram-positive bacteria may play a role in the development of NEC in preterm infants [61].

(16) In 2011, *Mai et al.* [62] compared the diversity of microbiota and prevalence of specific bacterial signatures in preterm infants (≤32 weeks of gestation or birth weight ≤1,250 g; 9 NEC cases and 9 gestation-matched controls) using

high-throughput 16S rRNA sequencing. Weekly stool samples (n = 110,021) were collected starting with the first stool and continued until discharge. Microbiota composition differed in control samples collected 1 week but not <72 h before the diagnosis of NEC. Between the 1-week and <72-h samples, Proteobacteria increased (34%), Firmicutes decreased (32%), and some of the molecular signatures were increased in NEC cases. One of the more frequently detected bacterial signatures ($p < 0.01$) matched closest to Gammaproteobacteria. Although this sequence was close to the Enterobacteriaceae family, it did not match any sequence in GenBank by >97%. Further data are required to confirm if this microbe contributes to the development of NEC [62].

(17) In 2009, *Wang et al.* [63] compared fecal microbiota in preterm infants who did (10 cases) versus those who did not (10 controls, including 4 twin pairs) develop NEC by 16S rRNA gene sequencing and terminal restriction fragment length polymorphism analysis. Gut microbiota showed low diversity in the samples from all infants. Infants with NEC showed a further decrease in diversity, increased abundance of Gammaproteobacteria, and a decrease in other bacterial species. They had received antibiotics for a longer duration prior to developing NEC. These findings support the role of a diminished diversity of the gut microbiome and prolonged exposure to antibiotics in the development of NEC [63].

Discussion

Overall, the current evidence indicates that in contrast to the healthy adult gut microbiota, the early postnatal gut microbiota of preterm infants is simple, very diverse, and dynamic, and plays an important role in the development of NEC [28]. Given the number of factors involved in shaping the early gut microbiota in preterm infants, including the mode of delivery, gestational and postnatal age, type of milk feeds, exposure to antibiotics in the early pre- and postnatal period, and exposure to gastric acid inhibitors, it is not surprising that the results of gut microbiota studies in preterm infants are difficult to interpret [64–69]. Differences in the methodology for assessing the gut microbiota further complicate the issue. However, experts point out that the results are mostly similar when diverse methods (e.g. culture-based or molecular methods) are used in the same study [69–75]. Investigators report that culture-based methods miss relatively few, if any, bacterial species when analyzing the early microbiota [76]. Most studies have assessed fecal microbiota, and results of mucosal biopsies and luminal content analysis seem to suggest/confirm the adequacy of fecal sampling [71, 77, 78].

Table 1. Summary of the studies included

First author	Method	NEC cases, *n*	Controls, *n*	Key findings
Warner et al. [47], 2016	16S rRNA Pyroseq	46	120	NEC was associated with significantly increased Gammaproteobacteria and decreased Negativicutes
Ward et al. [48], 2016	16S rRNA, DSMSA	27	89	Colonization with uropathogenic *Escherichia coli* was a risk factor for NEC and subsequent mortality; the strains included ST69, ST73, ST95, ST127, ST131, and ST144
Heida et al. [49], 2016	16S rRNA	11	22	Significantly increased presence and abundance of *Clostridium perfringens* and *Bacteroides dorei* in meconium in cases vs. controls; postmeconium samples: abundance of staphylococci negatively associated with NEC; *C. perfringens* more prevalent in NEC cases
Hourigan et al. [50], 2016	16S rRNA	1[a]	1[a]	Decreased bacterial diversity and increased Proteobacteria in the week preceding the signs of NEC in the twin who developed the illness
Cortese et al. [51], 2016	16S rRNA, qPCR	–	–	Microbial colonization may alter epigenetic signatures of the immature gut establishing inflammatory changes and compromising barrier properties predisposing to NEC
Abdulkadir et al. [52], 2016	16S rRNA, qPCR	10	10	No significant difference in TBL in cases vs. controls; no significant temporal changes in TBL within cases before vs. after NEC diagnosis, and in controls
Cassir et al. [53], 2015	16S rRNA, Pyroseq, qPCR	15	15	*Clostridium butyricum* specifically associated with NEC using molecular and culture-based methods
Zhou et al. [54], 2015	16S rRNA	10	26	The specific pathogens (e.g., Gammaproteobacteria) associated with NEC may vary by the infant's postnatal age at onset of NEC
McMurtry et al. [55], 2015	16S rRNA, Pyroseq, qPCR	21	74	Microbial diversity and Clostridia abundance and prevalence decreased with increasing severity of NEC
Raveh-Sadka et al. [56], 2015	16S rRNA	5	5	Strains colonizing each infant in the unit were distinct, and none was common to infants who developed NEC; the paucity of shared gut colonizers suggested significant barriers to the spread of bacteria among infants
Sim et al. [57], 2015	16S rRNA, FAFLP typing	12	44	A clostridial OTU was overabundant in samples from infants with NEC before diagnosis; culture confirmed *C. perfringens* type A; FAFLP typing showed that no isolates were identical; samples from NEC cases before diagnosis without profuse *C. perfringens* showed an overabundance of *Klebsiella* OTU
Brower-Sinning et al. [58], 2014	16S rRNA	16	10	TBL was higher in NEC samples; both NEC and non-NEC samples showed high interindividual variability and an abundance of opportunistic pathogens; NEC samples showed an abundance of strict anaerobes and a decreased diversity of the bacterial community and no uniform pattern of microbial colonization
Claud et al. [59], 2013	16S rRNA	5	5	Gut microbiome differed in cases vs. controls, starting from 3 weeks before diagnosis of NEC; the majority of the differentially abundant genes in cases were associated with carbohydrate metabolism and mapped to the Enterobacteriaceae family

Table 1. Continued

First author	Method	NEC cases, *n*	Controls, *n*	Key findings
Normann et al. [60], 2013	Bar-coded Pyroseq	10	20	Gut microbiota was dominated by *Enterococcus*, Bacillales, and Enterobacteriaceae in cases; high relative abundance of Bacillales and Enterobacteriaceae preceded the diagnosis of NEC; *Enterococcus* dominated gut flora in control samples; a low diversity of gut microbiota without significant differences between NEC vs. controls
Smith et al. [61], 2012	PCR-DGGE	21	142	Gram-positive bacteria predominant in NEC samples; control group had mixed flora of gram-positive and -negative bacteria
Mai et al. [62], 2011	High-throughput 16S rRNA	9	9	Between the 1-week and <72-h samples, Proteobacteria increased, Firmicutes decreased, and some of the molecular signatures were increased in NEC cases; one of the more frequently detected bacterial signatures matched closest to Gammaproteobacteria
Wang et al. [63], 2009	16S rRNA, TRFLPA	10	10	Gut microbiota showed low diversity in cases and controls; infants with NEC showed a further decrease in diversity, increased abundance of Gammaproteobacteria, and a decrease in other bacterial species

The study by Cortese et al. [51] was an experimental study. DSMSA, deep shotgun metagenomic sequence analysis; FAFLP, fluorescent amplified fragment length polymorphism; OTU, operational taxonomic unit; Pyroseq, pyrosequencing; DGGE, denaturing gradient gel electrophoresis; qPCR, quantitative polymerase chain reaction; TBL, total bacterial load; TRFLPA, terminal restriction fragment length polymorphism analysis.
[a] Pair of twins discordant for NEC.

Further research is required to understand the significance of temporal changes in the gut microbiome in the early postnatal period, specific bacterial molecular signatures, and the relative abundance of Gammaproteobacteria as well as the paucity of strict anaerobic bacteria that precede NEC in preterm infants. The possibility that changes in the gut microbiota may be a consequence rather than a cause of NEC in preterm infants also needs to be considered [79]. Warner and Tarr [80] have recently reviewed studies [22, 47–49, 54–58, 62] in this field that used 16S rRNA/metagenomic sequencing on at least 100 stools from ≥100 matched controls. Assessing the reproducibility of previous findings (Table 1) in large prospective studies is important. Finally, issues with sample processing, the choice of the PCR primer, laboratory contamination, and differences in DNA extraction methods need to be considered in interpreting results of bacteriological assessments [81–83].

Disclosure Statement

The author declares no potential source of conflict of interest in relation to this work.

References

1 Neu J, Walker WA: Necrotizing enterocolitis. N Engl J Med 2011;364:255–264.
2 Lin PW, Stoll BJ: Necrotising enterocolitis. Lancet 2006;368:1271–1283.
3 Lin HC, Chang JH, Chung M-Y, Lin HC: Prevention of necrotizing enterocolitis in preterm very low birth weight infants: is it feasible? J Formos Med Assoc 2014;113:e490–e497.
4 Gagliardi L, Bellù R, et al; Network Neonatale Lombardo: Necrotising enterocolitis in very low birth weight infants in Italy: incidence and non-nutritional risk factors. J Pediatr Gastroenterol Nutr 2008;47:206–210.
5 Rowe MI, Reblock KK, Kurkchubasche AG, Healey PJ: Necrotizing enterocolitis in the extremely low birth weight infant. J Pediatr Surg 1994;29:987–990; discussion 990–991.
6 Salhab WA, Perlman JM, Silver L, Broyels SR: Necrotizing enterocolitis and neurodevelopmental outcome in extremely low birth weight infants <1,000 g. J Perinatol 2004;24: 534–540.
7 Walsh MC, Kliegman RM: Necrotising enterocolitis: treatment based on staging criteria. Pediatr Clin North Am 1986;33:179–201.
8 Sheng Q, Lv Z, Xu W, et al: Short-term surgical outcomes of preterm infants with necrotizing enterocolitis: a single-center experience. Medicine (Baltimore) 2016;95:e4379.
9 Henry MC, Moss RL: Surgical therapy for necrotizing enterocolitis: bringing evidence to the bedside. Semin Pediatr Surg 2005;14: 180–190.
10 Jones KD, Howarth LJ: Intestinal failure following necrotizing enterocolitis: a clinical approach. Early Hum Dev 2016;97:29–32.
11 Wadhawan R, Oh W, et al; NICHD Neonatal Research Network. Neurodevelopmental outcomes of extremely low birth weight infants with spontaneous intestinal perforation or surgical necrotizing enterocolitis. J Perinatol 2014;34:64–70.
12 Pike K, Brocklehurst P, Jones D, et al: Outcomes at 7 years for babies who developed neonatal necrotising enterocolitis: the ORACLE Children Study. Arch Dis Child Fetal Neonatal Ed 2012;97:F318–F322.
13 Schulzke SM, Deshpande GC, Patole SK: Neurodevelopmental outcomes of very low-birth-weight infants with necrotizing enterocolitis: a systematic review of observational studies. Arch Pediatr Adolesc Med 2007;161: 583–590.
14 Blakely ML, Lally KP, et al; NEC Subcommittee of the NICHD Neonatal Research Network: Postoperative outcomes of extremely low birth-weight infants with necrotizing enterocolitis or isolated intestinal perforation: a prospective cohort study by the NICHD Neonatal Research Network. Ann Surg 2005;241: 984–989; discussion 989–994.
15 Bisquera JA, Cooper TR, Berseth CL: Impact of necrotizing enterocolitis on length of stay and hospital charges in very low birth weight infants. Pediatrics 2002;109:423–428.
16 Torrazza RM, Li N, Neu J: Decoding the enigma of necrotizing enterocolitis in premature infants. Pathophysiology 2014;21:21–27.
17 Choi YY: Necrotizing enterocolitis in newborns: update in pathophysiology and newly emerging therapeutic strategies. Korean J Pediatr 2014;57:505–513.
18 Nanthakumar N, Meng D, Goldstein AM, et al: The mechanism of excessive intestinal inflammation in necrotizing enterocolitis: an immature innate immune response. PLoS One 2011;6:e17776.
19 Nanthakumar NN, Fusunyan RD, Sanderson I, Walker WA: Inflammation in the developing human intestine: a possible pathophysiologic contribution to necrotizing enterocolitis. Proc Natl Acad Sci U S A 2000;97: 6043–6048.
20 Emami CN, Petrosyan M, Giuliani S, et al: Role of the host defense system and intestinal microbial flora in the pathogenesis of necrotizing enterocolitis. Surg Infect (Larchmt) 2009;10:407–417.
21 Torrazza RM, Neu J: The altered gut microbiome and necrotizing enterocolitis. Clin Perinatol 2013;40:93–108.
22 Torrazza RM, Ukhanova M, Wang X, et al: Intestinal microbial ecology and environmental factors affecting necrotizing enterocolitis. PLoS One 2013;8:e83304.
23 Egan CE, Sodhi CP, Good M, et al: Toll-like receptor 4-mediated lymphocyte influx induces neonatal necrotizing enterocolitis. J Clin Invest 2016;126:495–508.

24 Guo S, Nighot M, Al-Sadi R, et al: Lipopolysaccharide regulation of intestinal tight junction permeability is mediated by TLR4 signal transduction pathway activation of FAK and MyD88. J Immunol 2015;195:4999–5010.
25 Afrazi A, Branca MF, Sodhi CP, et al: Toll-like receptor 4-mediated endoplasmic reticulum stress in intestinal crypts induces necrotizing enterocolitis. J Biol Chem 2014;289: 9584–9599.
26 Lu P, Sodhi CP, Hackam DJ: Toll-like receptor regulation of intestinal development and inflammation in the pathogenesis of necrotizing enterocolitis. Pathophysiology 2014;21: 81–93.
27 Elgin TG, Kern SL, McElroy SJ: Development of the neonatal intestinal microbiome and its association with necrotizing enterocolitis. Clin Ther 2016;38:706–715.
28 Grishin A, Bowling J, Bell B, et al: Roles of nitric oxide and intestinal microbiota in the pathogenesis of necrotizing enterocolitis. J Pediatr Surg 2016;51:13–17.
29 Coggins SA, Wynn JL, Weitkamp J-H: Infectious causes of necrotizing enterocolitis. Clin Perinatol 2015;42:133–154.
30 Zvizdic Z, Heljic S, Firdus A, et al: Relationship of nosocomial infections with the development of necrotizing enterocolitis in preterm infants. Mater Sociomed 2014;26:4–6.
31 Pineda LC, Hornik CP, Seed PC, et al: Association between positive urine cultures and necrotizing enterocolitis in a large cohort of hospitalized infants. Early Hum Dev 2015;91: 583–586.
32 Gupta S, Morris JG Jr, Panigrahi P, et al: Endemic necrotizing enterocolitis: lack of association with a specific infectious agent. Pediatr Infect Dis J 1994;13:728–734.
33 Peter CS, Feuerhahn M, Bohnhorst B, et al: Necrotising enterocolitis: is there a relationship to specific pathogens? Eur J Pediatr 1999;158:67–70.
34 Siu YK, Ng PC, Fung SC, et al: Double blind, randomised, placebo controlled study of oral vancomycin in prevention of necrotising enterocolitis in preterm, very low birthweight infants. Arch Dis Child Fetal Neonatal Ed 1998;79:F105–F109.
35 Grylack LJ, Scanlon JW: Oral gentamicin therapy in the prevention of neonatal necrotizing enterocolitis. A controlled double-blind trial. Am J Dis Child 1978;132:1192–1194.
36 Egan EA, Mantilla G, Nelson RM, Eitzman DV: A prospective controlled trial of oral kanamycin in the prevention of neonatal necrotizing enterocolitis. J Pediatr 1976;89:467–470.
37 Leach ST, Lui K, Naing Z, et al: Multiple opportunistic pathogens, but not pre-existing inflammation, may be associated with necrotizing enterocolitis. Dig Dis Sci 2015;60: 3728–3734.
38 Guner YS, Franklin AL, Chokshi NK, et al: P-glycoprotein induction by breast milk attenuates intestinal inflammation in experimental necrotizing enterocolitis. Lab Invest 2011;91:1668–1679.
39 Caubilla-Barron J, Hurrell E, Townsend S, et al: Genotypic and phenotypic analysis of *Enterobacter sakazakii* strains from an outbreak resulting in fatalities in a neonatal intensive care unit in France. J Clin Microbiol 2007;45: 3979–3985.
40 Franco AA, Hu L, Grim CJ, et al: Characterization of putative virulence genes on the related RepFIB plasmids harbored by *Cronobacter* spp. Appl Environ Microbiol 2011;77: 3255–3267.
41 Mange JP, Stephan R, Borel N, et al: Adhesive properties of *Enterobacter sakazakii* to human epithelial and brain microvascular endothelial cells. BMC Microbiol 2006;6:58.
42 Townsend S, Hurrell E, Forsythe S: Virulence studies of *Enterobacter sakazakii* isolates associated with a neonatal intensive care unit outbreak. BMC Microbiol 2008;8:64.
43 Hunter CJ, Petrosyan M, Ford HR, Prasadarao NV: *Enterobacter sakazakii*: an emerging pathogen in infants and neonates. Surg Infect (Larchmt) 2008;9:533–539.
44 Hunter CJ, Singamsetty VK, Chokshi NK: *Enterobacter sakazakii* enhances epithelial cell injury by inducing apoptosis in a rat model of necrotizing enterocolitis. J Infect Dis 2008;198:586–593.
45 Chokshi NK, Guner YS, Hunter CJ, et al: The role of nitric oxide in intestinal epithelial injury and restitution in neonatal necrotizing enterocolitis. Semin Perinatol 2008;32:92–99.
46 Hunter CJ, Williams M, Petrosyan M: *Lactobacillus bulgaricus* prevents intestinal epithelial cell injury caused by *Enterobacter sakazakii*-induced nitric oxide both in vitro and in the newborn rat model of necrotizing enterocolitis. Infect Immun 2009;77:1031–1043.

47 Warner BB, Deych E, Zhou Y, et al: Gut bacteria dysbiosis and necrotising enterocolitis in very low birth weight infants: a prospective case-control study. Lancet 2016;387:1928–1936.
48 Ward DV, Scholz M, Zolfo M, et al: Metagenomic sequencing with strain-level resolution implicates uropathogenic *E. coli* in necrotizing enterocolitis and mortality in preterm infants. Cell Rep 2016;14:2912–2924.
49 Heida FH, van Zoonen AG, Hulscher JB, et al: A necrotizing enterocolitis-associated gut microbiota is present in the meconium: results of a prospective study. Clin Infect Dis 2016;62:863–870.
50 Hourigan SK, Ta A, Wong WS, et al: The microbiome in necrotizing enterocolitis: a case report in twins and mini review. Clin Ther 2016;38:747–753.
51 Cortese R, Lu L, Yu Y, et al: Epigenome-microbiome crosstalk: a potential new paradigm influencing neonatal susceptibility to disease. Epigenetics 2016;11:205–215.
52 Abdulkadir B, Nelson A, Skeath T, et al: Stool bacterial load in preterm infants with necrotising enterocolitis. Early Hum Dev 2016;95:1–2.
53 Cassir N, Benamar S, Khalil JB, et al: *Clostridium butyricum* strains and dysbiosis linked to necrotizing enterocolitis in preterm neonates. Clin Infect Dis 2015;61:1107–1115.
54 Zhou Y, Shan G, Sodergren E, et al: Longitudinal analysis of the premature infant intestinal microbiome prior to necrotizing enterocolitis: a case-control study. PLoS One 2015;10:e0118632.
55 McMurtry VE, Gupta RW, Tran L, et al: Bacterial diversity and Clostridia abundance decrease with increasing severity of necrotizing enterocolitis. Microbiome 2015;3:11.
56 Raveh-Sadka T, Thomas BC, Singh A, et al: Gut bacteria are rarely shared by co-hospitalized premature infants, regardless of necrotizing enterocolitis development. eLife 2015;4:e05477.
57 Sim K, Shaw AG, Randell P, et al: Dysbiosis anticipating necrotizing enterocolitis in very premature infants. Clin Infect Dis 2015;60:389–397.
58 Brower-Sinning R, Zhong D, Good M, et al: Mucosa-associated bacterial diversity in necrotizing enterocolitis. PLoS One 2014;9:e105046.
59 Claud EC, Keegan KP, Brulc JM, et al: Bacterial community structure and functional contributions to emergence of health or necrotizing enterocolitis in preterm infants. Microbiome 2013;1:20.
60 Normann E, Fahlén A, Engstrand L, Lilja HE: Intestinal microbial profiles in extremely preterm infants with and without necrotizing enterocolitis. Acta Paediatr 2013;102:129–136.
61 Smith B, Bodé S, Skov TH, et al: Investigation of the early intestinal microflora in premature infants with/without necrotizing enterocolitis using two different methods. Pediatr Res 2012;71:115–120.
62 Mai V, Young CM, Ukhanova M, et al: Fecal microbiota in premature infants prior to necrotizing enterocolitis. PLoS One 2011;6:e20647.
63 Wang Y, Hoenig JD, Malin KJ, et al: 16S rRNA gene-based analysis of fecal microbiota from preterm infants with and without necrotizing enterocolitis. ISME J 2009;3:944–954.
64 Kuppala VS, Meinzen-Derr J, Morrow AL, Schibler KR: Prolonged initial empirical antibiotic treatment is associated with adverse outcomes in premature infants. J Pediatr 2011;159:720–725.
65 Cotten CM, Taylor S, et al: NICHD Neonatal Research Network: Prolonged duration of initial empirical antibiotic treatment is associated with increased rates of necrotizing enterocolitis and death for extremely low birth weight infants. Pediatrics 2009;123:58–66.
66 Weintraub AS, Ferrara L, Deluca L, et al: Antenatal antibiotic exposure in preterm infants with necrotizing enterocolitis. J Perinatol 2012;32:705–709.
67 Kenyon SL, Taylor DJ, Tarnow-Mordi W; ORACLE Collaborative Group: Broad-spectrum antibiotics for preterm, prelabour rupture of fetal membranes: the ORACLE I randomised trial. ORACLE Collaborative Group. Lancet 2001;357:979–988.
68 More K, Athalye-Jape G, Rao S, Patole S: Association of inhibitors of gastric acid secretion and higher incidence of necrotizing enterocolitis in preterm very low-birth-weight infants. Am J Perinatol 2013;30:849–856.
69 Arboleya S, Binetti A, Salazar N: Establishment and development of intestinal microbiota in preterm neonates. FEMS Microbiol Ecol 2011;79:763–772.

70 Hallstrom M, Eerola E, Vuento R, et al: Effects of mode of delivery and necrotising enterocolitis on the intestinal microflora in preterm infants. Eur J Clin Microbiol Infect Dis 2004;23:463–470.
71 Hoy CM, Wood CM, Hawkey PM, Puntis JW: Duodenal microflora in very-low-birth-weight neonates and relation to necrotizing enterocolitis. J Clin Microbiol 2000;38:4539–4547.
72 Jacquot A, Neveu D, Aujoulat F: Dynamics and clinical evolution of bacterial gut microflora in extremely premature patients. J Pediatr 2011;158:390–396.
73 Millar MR, Linton CJ, Cade A, et al: Application of 16S rRNA gene PCR to study bowel flora of preterm infants with and without necrotizing enterocolitis. J Clin Microbiol 1996;34:2506–2510.
74 Rouge C, Goldenberg O, Ferraris L, et al: Investigation of the intestinal microbiota in preterm infants using different methods. Anaerobe 2010;16:362–370.
75 Schwiertz A, Gruhl B, Löbnitz M, et al: Development of the intestinal bacterial composition in hospitalized preterm infants in comparison with breast-fed, full-term infants. Pediatr Res 2003;54:393–393.
76 Magne F, Abély M, Boyer F, et al: Low species diversity and high interindividual variability in faeces of preterm infants as revealed by sequences of 16S rRNA genes and PCR-temporal temperature gradient gel electrophoresis profiles. FEMS Microbiol Ecol 2006;57: 128–138.
77 Blakey JL, Lubitz L, Barnes GL, et al: Development of gut colonisation in pre-term neonates. J Med Microbiol 1982;15:519–529.
78 Nakayama M, Yajima M, Hatano S, et al: Intestinal adherent bacteria and bacterial translocation in breast-fed and formula-fed rats in relation to susceptibility to infection. Pediatr Res 2003;54:364–371.
79 Stewart CJ, Cummings SP: Gut bacteria and necrotizing enterocolitis: cause or effect? Trends Microbiol 2015;23:332–333.
80 Warner BB, Tarr PI: Necrotizing enterocolitis and preterm infant gut bacteria. Semin Fetal Neonatal Med 2016;21:394–399
81 Walker AW, Martin JC, Scott P, et al: 16S rRNA gene-based profiling of the human infant gut microbiota is strongly influenced by sample processing and PCR primer choice. Microbiome 2015;3:26.
82 Salter SJ, Cox MJ, Turek EM, et al: Reagent and laboratory contamination can critically impact sequence-based microbiome analyses. BMC Biol 2014;12:87.
83 Kennedy NA, Walker AW, Berry SH, et al: The impact of different DNA extraction kits and laboratories upon the assessment of human gut microbiota composition by 16S rRNA gene sequencing. PLoS One 2014; 9:e88982.

Isolauri E, Sherman PM, Walker WA (eds): Intestinal Microbiome: Functional Aspects in Health and Disease. Nestlé Nutr Inst Workshop Ser, vol 88, pp 95–105, (DOI: 10.1159/000455217)
Nestec Ltd., Vevey/S. Karger AG., Basel, © 2017

Microbiota and Obesity

Erika Isolauri

Department of Pediatrics and Adolescent Medicine, Turku University Hospital, and Department of Clinical Sciences, Faculty of Medicine, University of Turku, Turku, Finland

Abstract

Obesity is globally the most prevalent nutritional disorder. Multifaceted therapeutic approaches are called for to halt the cascade from neonatal adiposity/high birth weight to childhood excessive weight gain/adult obesity with comorbidities. Recent experimental and clinical data provide one new target for interventions aiming to close this vicious circle: the microbiota. An aberrant gut microbiota, dysbiosis, induces immune and metabolic disturbances both locally and, consequent upon impaired gut barrier function, also systemic low-grade inflammation, which is causally linked to insulin resistance. The gut microecology could thus fill the gap between energy intake and expenditure by processing nutrients and regulating their access to and storage in the body, producing chemicals of hormonal nature and controlling the secretion of proinflammatory mediators locally and systemically. Conversely, being highly sensitive to environmental impacts, particularly to early feeding, the compositional development of the gut microbiota may prove the target of choice in efforts to reduce the risk of obesity. It has been demonstrated that a lower number of bifidobacteria precedes the development of obesity, and a dearth of butyrate-producing bacteria and an overall richness of bacteria increase the risk of metabolic disease; moreover, recognition that practices known to disrupt the early gut microbiota, e.g., cesarean section delivery and antibiotic exposure, contribute to obesity, encourages to pursue this line of research.

Obesity – The Epidemic

Concurrently with important advances in medicine, the burden of obesity has become a plague of our times; whether the link is causal remains elusive. Obesity is the common denominator of diet-related chronic disorders such as cardiovascular disease and diabetes, but also chronic inflammatory and allergic diseases. Indeed, overweight and obesity can be seen as belonging to the family of noncommunicable diseases sharing common environmental risk factors and immunologic features, which frequently coexist and constitute a threat to human well-being. Somewhat belatedly, the list of entwining conditions now extends to mood and brain, wired to the gut by means of bidirectional exchange of endocrine and immune and neural signals.

Obesity is globally the most prevalent nutritional disorder among children. Two decades ago, the World Health Organization declared obesity a global epidemic [1]. The term defines groups of cases resembling each other and, secondly, groups of different diseases occurring in the same place or in the same season and sometimes spreading "on *(epi)* the people *(demos)*", in contrast to *nosos*, a term used to describe diseases at individual level [2].

The NCD Risk Factor Collaboration found that the mean age-corrected body mass index (kg/m^2) has continued to increase in men and women alike, exceeding 24 in both, in 200 countries and territories between 1975 and 2014 [3]. During this period, the risk of becoming obese was higher than that of being underweight. The obesity epidemic is thus a moving target, and a solution is both challenging and urgent. The velocity of propagation of the epidemic is high in children and young adults of reproductive age with the potential to transmit the propensity to the next generation [4]. The risk of escalation of the problem should be given high priority in health policy, and prevention is better than cure.

The Microbiota: Origin and Potential in Reducing the Obesity Risk

The hygiene hypothesis suggests that environmental changes in the industrialized world have led to reduced microbial contact at an early age and thus contributed to the epidemic of atopic disease [reviewed in 5]. In 1976, Gerrard et al. [5] found an inverse relationship between the incidence of infections and atopic disease and concluded that a relative freedom from diseases due to viruses, bacteria, and helminths caused the latter. Again, in 1989, Strachan [6] detected an inverse correlation between family size and the prevalence of allergic rhinitis and suggested that infections acquired from older siblings might confer protection against the development of atopic disease.

An extended version of the hygiene hypothesis has since been introduced [7] to underscore the intimate interrelationship between the immune system and the microbiota and link their united forces to the theory of developmental origins of health and disease [8]. Accordingly, the risk of noncommunicable diseases is heightened if the environmental conditions after birth differ from those experienced by the fetus during pregnancy. Epidemiological data corroborate the importance of stable pre- and postnatal nutrition: restricted in utero

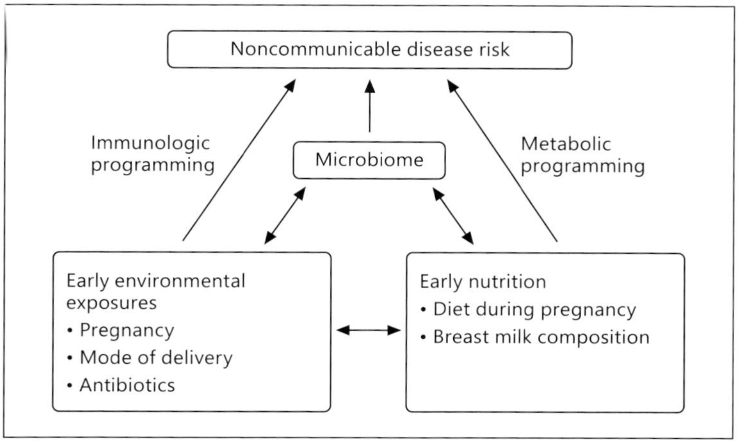

Fig. 1. A schematic presentation of the proposed relationship between the gut microbiota and early environment and nutrition, which underlie the risk of noncommunicable diseases in childhood.

nutrition followed by the abundant supply of nutrition in the Western lifestyle increases susceptibility to metabolic disorders [9]. Clinical evidence, again, points to both maternal under- and overnutrition in pregnancy as equally inductive of an obesity risk in the child [reviewed in 4, 10].

This concept may be extrapolated from nutrition to the host-microbe interaction. Undeniably, modern techniques have generated a microbiome renaissance, and the forgotten organ is now given the attention its size and impact deserves, particularly during the critical period of programming. In fact, microbe contact in the perinatal period represents the most massive antigen exposure educating the physiological adaptation processes to the anticipated postnatal environment. The newborn lacking an age-appropriate and environment-adjusted microbe contact optimal for timely maturation of the immune, metabolic, and neural regulatory systems may be predisposed to develop allergic disease, chronic inflammatory conditions, and obesity (Fig. 1).

The extended hygiene hypothesis calls for a prudent review of clinical practices, which may interfere with the healthy host-microbe interaction during the critical period within which, according to the developmental origins of the health and disease theory, the immune and metabolic phenotype is consolidated (Fig. 1). These practices include delivery by cesarean section and antibiotic use. Elective cesarean section accompanied by antibiotic treatment hinders the establishment of the gut microbiota more or less transiently but nonetheless carries long-term clinical consequences manifested as immune-inflammatory conditions as well as obesity [11]. The impact of maternal obesity may still constitute a confounder here. A recent systematic review and meta-analysis, however, has demonstrated that cesarean section exerts an independent effect on obesity in children, even when the results were adjusted for maternal prepregnancy weight [12]. Epidemiological data linking early antibiotic exposure to a later obesity risk are more conflicting. One potential explanation might be sought in the limitations of register data, retrospective or large cohort studies, or epidemiological methods of evaluating interactions with detailed host characteristics such as diet, health, and prevailing gut microbiota composition. Indeed, antibiotic exposure was shown to exert distinct effects in infants of mothers with a high pre-pregnancy body mass index as compared to those of normal-weight mothers; antibiotic exposure reduced the risk in the former but increased it in the latter [13].

In point of fact, the rate of cesarean section delivery exceeds the WHO recommendation for nonmedical reasons, and the cumulative trend seems to continue [14]. Conversely, the rate of breastfeeding fails to reach current recommendations; breastfeeding guides the healthy compositional development of gut microbiota postnatally.

Finally, the contribution of mother's health, weight, and weight gain during pregnancy to the metabolic health and disease risk of the child is recognized as being to a degree determined by the maternal gut and breast milk microbiota [11]. Indeed, the composition of the gut microbiota through pregnancy and within breast milk is not standard, but evinces marked individual variation [15]. These sources provide the inoculum for the establishment of the gut microbiota in the newborn. Different routes may communicate aberrancies in the mother's microbiota composition during pregnancy, at delivery via microbes in the mother's birth canal, and in close contact with the mother and her immediate environment after delivery [reviewed in 4].

One attractive idea arising from the unified hypothesis, the extended hygiene hypothesis linked to the developmental origins of health and disease theory, is modification of the maternal gut microbiota during pregnancy and the perinatal period, as well as the breast milk microbiota. Promoting a balanced host-microbe interaction may aid in attuning the child's gut microbiota to age and reprogramming the risk of chronic inflammatory conditions, including obesity.

Microbiota Functions in Metabolic Health

In light of the energy balance equation, obesity development appears straightforward: energy intake exceeds that expended. Indeed, the energy nutrients consumed excessively in the current sedentary Western lifestyle has been seen as the source of the obesity epidemic. Replacement of energy nutrients, however, by noncaloric substitutes has not provided a solution but may indeed have contributed to the obesity epidemic, emphasizing the multilayered mechanisms of nutrition-related conditions in humans. Simultaneously, the complex collection of the human gut microbiota has failed to adapt to the abundance of modern dietary preferences: a diet rich in fat, sugar, and protein and low in fiber. In fact, the task of the gut microbiota, an instrumental element of host defense, is strengthening of the gut barrier functions, competitive exclusion of pathogens, and alleviation of the intestinal inflammatory response (possibly for the purpose of resisting ancient food-borne infections), and concomitantly aiding in energy extraction and storage from the diet (conceivably to adjust to times of food shortage).

Recent scientific advances tend to challenge earlier reasoning that the gut microbiota functions merely as a barrier component efficient in assimilating antigens encountered by the enteral route. Experimental studies demonstrate that the immune and metabolic deviations involved in obesity may not derive linearly from dietary intake but rather from gut microbiota modifications induced by the diet [reviewed in 4]. Hence, notwithstanding incomplete evidence from clinical intervention studies thus far, the composition of the gut microbiota may be taken to represent a strategic contributor to obesity as it pertains to excessive energy intake from an unhealthy diet and disproportionate storage of energy owing to sedentary behavior.

Gut Microbiota and Obesity Epidemic: Cause, Consequence, or Mechanism?

Scientific interest in the potential causative role of the gut microbiota in obesity was attracted by the demonstration that a distinctive gut microbiota composition prevails in obese individuals, with adjustments following weight gain or weight loss [16]. In the same vein, aberrant compositional development of the gut microbiota is documented during breastfeeding in infants in whom overweight development was documented, i.e. gut microbiota deviation precedes obesity [17]. Further support for the conception of microbiota involvement in obesity is obtained by epidemiological data linking known causes of gut microbiota disturbance early in life, namely cesarean section delivery and antibiotic exposure, to the subsequent development of overweight and obesity [reviewed in 4]. Experimental studies, again, have improved our understanding of mechanisms and causality in this context. Taken together, these elements markedly reinforce the hypothesis that modification of gut microbial communities might offer a strategy applicable to obesity management [18].

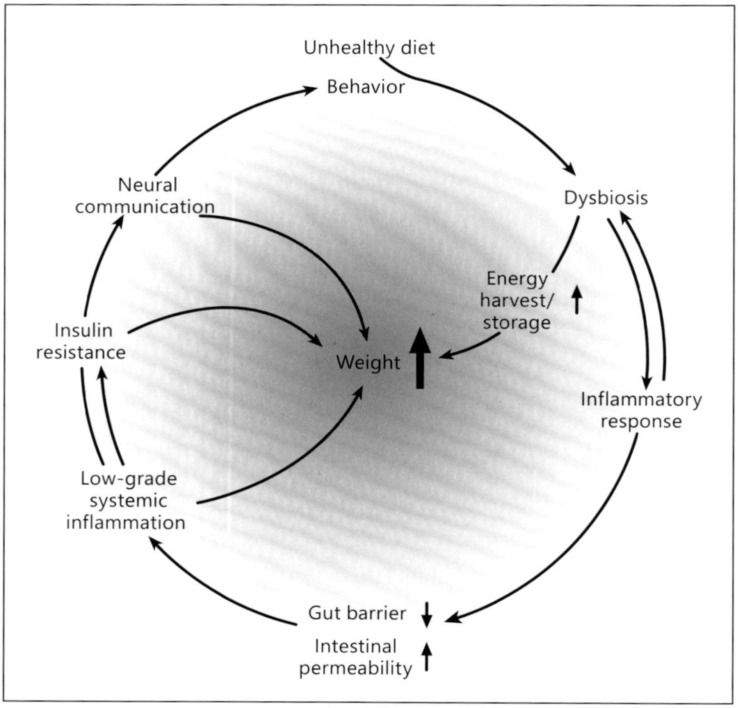

Fig. 2. The vicious circle of obesity.

The Western diet with its high-fat and -energy content has been associated with reduced gut microbiota diversity and perturbed composition, dysbiosis, an imbalance in the taxonomic composition of the gut microbiota. The gut microbiota impacts on metabolism by retrieving nutrients otherwise inaccessible to the host (Fig. 2). Experimental studies have provided evidence that specific gut microbiota profiles facilitate the extraction of calories from the diet and their storage in the host adipose tissue [19]. These phenomena have been shown to act simultaneously. Dysbiosis may increase energy efficiency via fermentation of nondigested food, thus providing more energy to the host; intestinal monosaccharide absorption and energy extraction as short-chain fatty acid (SCFA) production, combined with subsequent stimulation of de novo synthesis of triglycerides in the liver, boost weight gain. Furthermore, dysbiosis could increase fatty acid storage in adipocytes by suppressing the fasting-induced adipose factor in the gut, which in turn increases enzyme lipoprotein lipase activity in adipocytes and enhances fat storage [19]. A balanced gut microbiota composition, again, protects against diet-induced obesity by inhibition of cellular energy-dependent protein kinase activation [20]. A third potential explanation lies in the association between SCFA signaling molecule activation and energy storage [21].

The role of SCFAs in enhancing energy efficiency may be more complex than initially anticipated. SCFAs may exert beneficial metabolic effects in adipose tissue and the liver and improve insulin sensitivity. A lower abundance of butyrate-producing bacteria has been associated with an increased metabolic disease risk in humans, as butyrate-producing microbes show an anti-inflammatory potential and alleviation of the metabolic disturbances of obesity. The effect of butyrate on the intestinal barrier is nonetheless paradoxical. Butyrate may promote gut barrier function at a low concentration, while a high concentration may have the opposite effect [22]. Equally, SCFA acetate, produced by specific bifidobacteria, promoted intestinal defense mediated by epithelial cells [reviewed in 23]. Enhanced production of acetate, a substrate to cholesterol and triglyceride synthesis, was observed in experimental animals fed a high-fat diet compared to counterparts on standard diets [24]. Further, acetate was documented to increase, firstly, ghrelin levels and thereby also drive the host to eat excessively, and, secondly, glucose-stimulated insulin secretion. Acetate administration centrally in the brain increased glucose-stimulated insulin secretion, while pancreatic stimulation by acetate failed to accomplish this effect.

Glucose-stimulated insulin secretion proved able to be induced in recipient animals by fecal transplantation from animals on a high-fat diet. Microbiota depletion, in contrast, suppressed acetate turnover and reduced ghrelin levels. SCFA propionate shows a potential to protect against inflammatory responses by lowering fatty acid levels in plasma and to improve host glucose metabolism, unlike SFCA acetate in this experiment model. This distinction points to the site of activation of the parasympathetic nervous system mediated by the vagus nerve: the peripheral nervous system in the case of propionate and the central nervous system in the case of acetate [24]. Indeed, recent proof of gut microbiota involvement in obesity derives from the gut-brain axis, a bi-directional communication between the central nervous system and the gut.

Over and above processing nutrients and regulating their access to and storage in the body, activated inflammatory pathways are a corollary to "obesogenic microbiota" (Fig. 2). Indeed, the demonstration of active inflammatory cascades in the ileum in response to a high-fat diet prior to the onset of obesity invites the notion that the low-grade inflammation of obesity may be initiated in the gut, and specifically by the gut microbiota, the presence of which is a prerequisite in the progression of inflammation. Elevated systemic exposure to lipopolysaccharide, an endotoxin released by gram-negative bacteria, characterizes this inflammatory tone, defined as "metabolic endotoxemia" [25]. Aided by dysbiosis-induced impairment in the gut barrier function, lipopolysaccharides are delivered to CD14 and toll-like receptor 4, and the ensuing production of preinflammatory cytokines aggravates glucose and insulin metabolism and contributes to the onset of overweight-associated pathologies, including type 2 diabetes, hypertension, hepatic steatosis, and dyslipidemia [reviewed in: 4, 23, 26]. Interestingly, dietary fatty acids, of which circulating levels are often increased in obesity, have previously been shown to induce insulin resistance through the same signaling pathways, linking the nutritional environment to the gut microecology within the innate immune regulation [23, 26].

Gut Microbiota Profiles Are Causally Linked to the Obesity Risk

The most plausible evidence of a causal relationship between dysbiosis and the obesity risk has been obtained from experimental studies demonstrating that gut microbiota transfer from an obese individual can produce the obese phenotype in the recipient [27, 28]. Colonization of germ-free mice with the gut microbiota from an obese mouse or human enables weight gain and fat mass accumulation in these animals, without altered dietary intake. In accordance with this line of experimental work, there are clinical case reports on the treatment of recurrent diarrhea caused by *Clostridium difficile* by fecal transplantation, which demonstrate the development of obesity, the donor metabolic type, in the recipient [29].

It needs to be acknowledged that current demonstrations are far from complete in identifying specific constituents within the "obesogenic microbiota" as causative offending agents in the vicious circle of obesity. Phylum-wide compositional patterns have been shown to differ between obese and lean individuals but with contradictory outcomes [16, 19, 30]. These include reduced microbial diversity and a shift in the relative abundance of *Bacteroidetes* and *Firmicutes* and a higher abundance of *Proteobacteria*. It must also be conceded that different methods and populations and continuously developing techniques hamper direct comparisons among studies.

Data are accumulating, however, to prove the necessary initial step of dysbiosis in obesity, when the gut microbiota is taken as one operator [18]. An important conclusion to be drawn from human studies is that the rate of acquisition of certain microbiota patterns appears crucial for the programming of later health [reviewed in 4]. For example, a lower abundance of bifidobacteria, with specific species present, during the period of exclusive breastfeeding in vaginally delivered infants devoid of antibiotic exposure may predict adiposity [4, 17]. Experimental findings tend to substantiate this clinical finding by connecting high numbers of bifidobacteria with normalization of the inflammatory status and improved glucose tolerance and glucose-induced insulin secretion [31].

Likewise, at an early age, differences in *Bacteroides* group colonization may indicate disadvantaged metabolic health later [32]. Undernourished children in developing countries have exhibited a younger gut microbiota profile than expected for their chronological age [reviewed in: 4, 33], while precocious maturation has been seen in overweight children [34]. Further, the meconium microbiota of infants born to mothers with diabetes mellitus resembles that of an adult diabetic [35]. In adolescents and adults, increased numbers of *Proteobacteria* have been considered characteristic of dysbiosis [reviewed in 18], while *Akkermansia muciniphila*, a member of the *Verrucomicrobia*, may typify control over inflammation and adipose tissue metabolism [36]. In pregnant women, an association between gut microbiota composition and nutritional status has been reported [37], and specifically a gut microbiota profile higher in numbers of *Bifidobacterium* appeared to provide protection against maternal overweight development. In view of the microbial inoculum provided by the fetomaternal interface, along with microbe contact during delivery and through lactation, this species in particular has attracted clinical research interest [reviewed in 4].

The ultimate goal of clinical research in this context is defining an age-specific gut microbiota endorsing healthy development, documented in children remaining healthy also in the long term and thereby providing a gold standard of healthy human microbiota in the environment studied. Linking such microbiota profiles to experimental models improves our understanding of the mechanisms of host-microbe interactions in health and disease. Such research also provides microbiota markers and tools to modulate deviant microbiota development in at-risk populations. It is then the task of clinical intervention studies, in well-characterized human populations, to provide the final proof of causality for nutritional recommendations to combat the obesity epidemic.

Disclosure Statement

The author declares that no financial or other conflict of interest exists in relation to the contents of the chapter.

References

1 Obesity: preventing and managing the global epidemic. Report of a WHO consultation. Geneva, 3–5 June 1997. World Health Organ Tech Rep Ser 2000;894:1–253.

2 Martin PMV, Martin-Granel E: 2,500-year evolution of the term epidemic. Emerg Infect Dis 2006;12:976–980.

3 NCD Risk Factor Collaboration (NCD-RisC): Trends in adult body-mass index in 200 countries from 1975 to 2014: a pooled analysis of 1698 population-based measurement studies with 19.2 million participants. Lancet 2016;387:1377–1396.

4 Isolauri E, Rautava S, Collado MC, Salminen S: Early microbe contact in defining child metabolic health and obesity risk; in Green LR, Hester RL (eds): Parental Obesity: Intergenerational Programming and Consequences. Physiology in Health and Disease. New York, Springer, 2016.
5 Gerrard JW, Geddes CA, Reggin PL, et al: Serum IgE levels in white and metis communities in Saskatchewan. Ann Allergy 1976;37: 91–100.
6 Strachan DP: Hay fever, hygiene, and household size. BMJ 1989;299:1259–1260.
7 Rautava S, Kalliomäki M, Isolauri E: New therapeutic strategy for combating the increasing burden of allergic disease: probiotics. A Nutrition, Allergy, Mucosal Immunology and Intestinal Microbiota (NAMI) Research Group report. J Allergy Clin Immunol 2005;116:31–37.
8 Barker DJ: The origins of the developmental origins theory. J Intern Med 2007;261:412–417.
9 Gluckman PD, Hanson MA, Cooper C, Thornburg KL: Effect of in utero and early-life conditions on adult health and disease. N Engl J Med 2008;359:61–73.
10 Fall CH: Evidence for intra-uterine programming of adiposity in later life. Ann Hum Biol 2011;38:410–428.
11 Rautava S, Luoto R, Salminen S, Isolauri E: Microbial contact during pregnancy, intestinal colonization and human disease. Nat Rev Gastroenterol Hepatol 2012;9:565–576.
12 Kuhle S, Tong OS, Woolcott CG: Association between caesarean section and childhood obesity: a systematic review and meta-analysis. Obes Rev 2015;16:295–303.
13 Ajslev TA, Andersen CS, Gamborg M, et al: Childhood overweight after establishment of the gut microbiota: the role of delivery mode, pre-pregnancy weight and early administration of antibiotics. Int J Obes (Lond) 2011;35: 522–529.
14 Miettinen R, Hermansson H, Merikukka M, et al: Mode of delivery – impact on risk of noncommunicable diseases. J Allergy Clin Immunol 2015;136:1398–1399.
15 Cabrera-Rubio R, Collado MC, Laitinen K, et al: The human milk microbiome changes over lactation and is shaped by maternal weight and mode of delivery. Am J Clin Nutr 2012;96:544–551.
16 Ley RE, Bäckhed F, Turnbaugh P, et al: Obesity alters gut microbial ecology. Proc Natl Acad Sci U S A 2005;102:11070–11075.
17 Kalliomäki M, Collado MC, Salminen S, Isolauri E: Early differences in fecal microbiota composition in children may predict overweight. Am J Clin Nutr 2008;87:534–538.
18 Zhao L: The gut microbiota and obesity: from correlation to causality. Nat Rev Microbiol 2013;11:639–647.
19 Bäckhed F, Ding H, Wang T, et al: The gut microbiota as an environmental factor that regulates fat storage. Proc Natl Acad Sci U S A 2004;101:15718–15723.
20 Bäckhed F, Manchester JK, Semenkovich CF, Gordon JI: Mechanisms underlying the resistance to diet-induced obesity in germ-free mice. Proc Natl Acad Sci U S A 2007;104: 979–984.
21 Samuel BS, Shaito A, Motoike T, et al: Effects of the gut microbiota on host adiposity are modulated by the short-chain fatty-acid binding G protein-coupled receptor, Gpr41. Proc Natl Acad Sci U S A 2008;105:16767–16772.
22 Peng L, He Z, Chen W, et al: Effects of butyrate on intestinal barrier function in a Caco-2 cell monolayer model of intestinal barrier. Pediatr Res 2007;61:37–41.
23 Kau AL, Ahern PP, Griffin NW, et al: Human nutrition, the gut microbiome and the immune system. Nature 2011;474:327–336.
24 Perry RJ, Peng L, Barry NA, et al: Acetate mediates a microbiome-brain-β-cell axis to promote metabolic syndrome. Nature 2016;534: 213–217.
25 Cani PD, Amar J, Iglesias MA, et al: Metabolic endotoxemia initiates obesity and insulin resistance. Diabetes 2007;56:1761–1772.
26 Greer RL, Morgum A, Shulzhenko N: Bridging immunity and lipid metabolism by gut microbiota. J Allergy Clin Immunol 2013; 132:253–262.
27 Cox LM, Yamanishi S, Sohn J, et al: Altering the intestinal microbiota during a critical developmental window has lasting metabolic consequences. Cell 2014;158:705–721.
28 Koren O, Goodrich JK, Cullender TC, et al: Host remodeling of the gut microbiome and metabolic changes during pregnancy. Cell 2012;150:470–480.
29 Alang N, Kelly CR: Weight gain after fecal microbiota transplantation. Open Forum Infect Dis 2015;2:ofv004.

30 Shin NR, Whon TW, Bae JW: Proteobacteria: microbial signature of dysbiosis in gut microbiota. Trends Biotechnol 2015;33:496–503.
31 Cani PD, Neyrinck AM, Fava F, et al: Selective increases of bifidobacteria in gut microflora improve high-fat-diet-induced diabetes in mice through a mechanism associated with endotoxaemia. Diabetologia 2007;50:2374–2383.
32 Scheepers, LE, Penders, J, Mbakwa, CA, et al: The intestinal microbiota composition and weight development in children: the KOALA Birth Cohort Study. Int J Obes (Lond) 2015; 39:16–25.
33 Subramanian S, Huq S, Yatsunenko T, et al: Persistent gut microbiota immaturity in malnourished Bangladeshi children. Nature 2014;510:417–421.
34 Dogra S, Sakwinska O, Soh SE, et al; GUSTO Study Group: Dynamics of infant gut microbiota are influenced by delivery mode and gestational duration and are associated with subsequent adiposity. MBio 2015;6:e02419-14.
35 Hu J, Nomura Y, Bashir A, et al: Diversified microbiota of meconium is affected by maternal diabetes status. PLoS One 2013; 8:e78257.
36 Schneeberger M, Everard A, Gómez-Valadés AG, et al: *Akkermansia muciniphila* inversely correlates with the onset of inflammation, altered adipose tissue metabolism and metabolic disorders during obesity in mice. Sci Rep 2015;5:16643.
37 Collado MC, Isolauri E, Laitinen K, Salminen S: Distinct composition of gut microbiota during pregnancy in overweight and normal-weight women. Am J Clin Nutr 2008;88:894–899.

Isolauri E, Sherman PM, Walker WA (eds): Intestinal Microbiome: Functional Aspects in Health and Disease. Nestlé Nutr Inst Workshop Ser, vol 88, pp 107–115, (DOI: 10.1159/000455219)
Nestec Ltd., Vevey/S. Karger AG., Basel, © 2017

Microbiota in Functional Gastrointestinal Disorders in Infancy: Implications for Management

Thomas R. Abrahamsson[a] • Richard Y. Wu[b] • Philip M. Sherman[b]

[a]Clinical and Experimental Medicine, Linkoping University, Linkoping, Sweden; [b]Research Institute, Hospital for Sick Children, University of Toronto, Toronto, ON, Canada

Abstract

The complex and diverse intestinal microbiome is recognized as important in promoting human health. An altered gut microflora, referred to as dysbiosis, is increasingly recognized as having an etiologic role in a variety of conditions, including functional gastrointestinal disorders: colic in infants and irritable bowel syndrome in older children. Probiotics are defined as live microorganisms that, if ingested in sufficient amounts, restore microbial homeostasis and have a benefit on health. Randomized controlled trials indicate that probiotics can be effective in a variety of intestinal conditions, including colic and irritable bowel syndrome. Probiotics may promote gut microbial diversity, but timing of the intervention appears crucial. Strain-specific effects on colonization resistance, epithelial barrier integrity, modulation of signal transduction, impacts on innate and adaptive immune responses, and effects on visceral hyperalgesia likely explain the observed variability in various probiotic strains. In the future, probiotics are likely to be chosen for use in a defined clinical setting based on underlying mechanism(s) of action. The precise component of the probiotic agent mediating observed effects is the subject of current research. Unresolved issues relate to optimal dosages, timing of ingestion, single versus combination formulations, maintenance of viability in storage, and the merits of employing probiotic-derived products.

Introduction

Colic is one of a series of conditions affecting babies during their first year of life that frequently calls the attention of health care providers (Table 1). As summarized in the recently published Rome IV criteria for functional gastrointestinal disorders (now also referred to as disorders of gut-brain interaction) across the

Table 1. Functional gastrointestinal disorders in the first year of life[1]

Colic
Functional constipation
Dyschezia
Functional diarrhea (variously referred to as chronic nonspecific diarrhea of infancy)
Regurgitation

[1] Adapted from: Benninga et al. [1].

life span, colic is defined by the manifestations of recurrent (>3 times/week) and protracted (>3 h/day) periods of irritability, crying, and fussiness that begins in otherwise healthy babies during the first few months of life [1]. These infants are developmentally normal and have a normal growth velocity for age. Symptoms usually occur in the afternoon or evening hours and can be alarming for parents and other caregivers, who are concerned about underlying causes of the apparent abdominal pain and discomfort. However, colic is a transient, developmental issue that generally resolves before 6 months of age, as the baby grows older. Alarming features that should trigger a search for other underlying causes include unexplained fever suggesting an occult urinary tract infection and suboptimal growth velocity. Even though colic has been considered as an extreme variation in normal patterns of infant fussiness, the symptoms can cause considerable distress for caregivers who seek effective and safe interventions to see the baby, and themselves, through the stressful transition period.

Evidence that the Gut Microbiome Is Altered in Functional Gastrointestinal Disorders

Studies indicate that intestinal microbial dysbiosis is a feature in both children [2] and adults [3] with irritable bowel syndrome (IBS). As with many studies related to the gut microbiota in other human conditions, the unanswered question is whether the gut dysbiosis is an underlying cause of intestinal symptoms of abdominal pain, bloating, and flatulence. Studies show that colonic biopsies and colonic washes taken from adults with IBS have higher proteolytic activity and greater pronociceptive activity in a murine model of visceral sensitivity than in biopsies and washes derived from the colons of healthy, asymptomatic controls [4]. The source of protease activity mediating the observed effects could well be luminal microbes. Intervention studies that impact the gut microbiota composition and/or diversity are another approach to consider whether there is a cause-effect relationship between the gut microbiome and symptoms that are consistent with IBS.

In a study in Dutch infants, reduced diversity in bacterial species was identified in fecal samples taken from infants who went on to develop colic versus

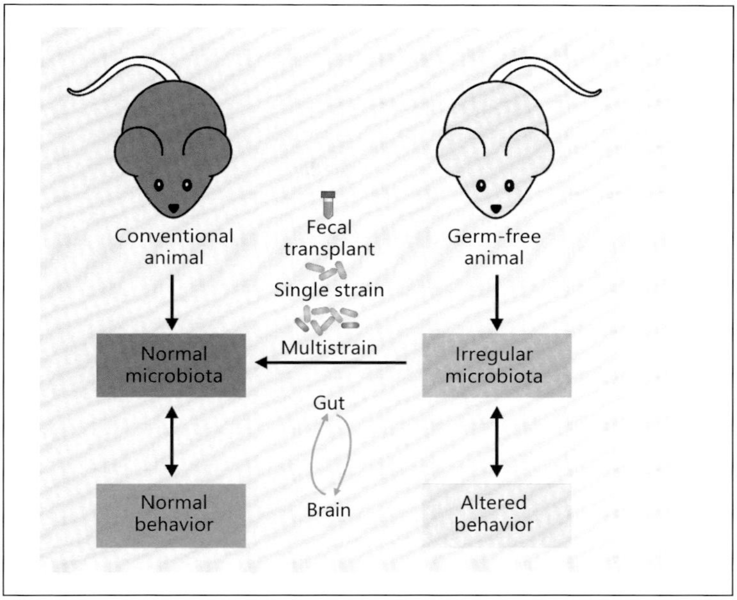

Fig. 1. Experimental evidence of the microbiome-gut-brain axis. In contrast to conventional animals, germ-free animals raised in pathogen-free environments are devoid of microorganisms in the intestinal tract. These animals have an altered immune system and behave differently than conventional animals. Reconstitution of the gut microbiome can be achieved via fecal transplants, cohousing of coprophagic animals, or using the targeted introduction of single or multiple strains of probiotics.

age-matched controls [5]. It should be noted that gender, birth weight, route of delivery, and duration of breastfeeding did not differ between the two study groups. In this study of 12 colicky babies and an equal number of asymptomatic subjects, microbial diversity was lower in stools obtained at 2 weeks of age in the study group with excessive crying. In particular, numbers of bifidobacteria and lactobacilli were reduced in babies who went on to develop colic. Since *Bifidobacterium* species and lactic acid-producing bacteria are frequently employed as probiotic preparations, there appears to be a rationale to use such agents to increase bacterial subpopulations that are reduced in numbers and thereby enhance gut microbial diversity. Validation of these findings in a larger number of infants in various parts of the world is now required.

Evidence that Altering the Gut Microbiota Impacts Symptoms in Irritable Bowel Syndrome

Increasing experimental and clinical evidence supports the existence of a bidirectional and modifiable microbiome-gut-brain axis [6]. As shown in Figure 1,

Table 2. Probiotic *Lactobacillus reuteri* DSM 17938 versus placebo in the management of infants with colic[1]

Reference No.	Country	Duration, days	Change in crying duration, min/day	95% confidence interval
14	Italy	28	–66.8	–78.4, –55.2
15	Italy	21	–125.0	–172.0, –78.0
16	Poland	21	–55.2	–60.2, –50.2
17	Australia	28	–11.0	–78.6, 100.6
18	China	28	–55.1	–55.1, –50.9
19	Canada	21	–39.8	–50.9, –28.7
Summary			–55.9	–64.4, –47.3**

** $p < 0.001$. [1] Adapted from: Harb et al. [12].

the behavior of germ-free mice differs from that observed of specific pathogen-free animals. Mice whose gut bacteria are disrupted by antibiotic treatment early in life had increased visceral sensitivity in adulthood, even though the composition of the gut microbiota had long been normalized [7]. Moreover, delivery of beneficial microbes (probiotics) has an impact on altering murine behavior that is mediated, at least in part, via vagal afferents because surgical vagotomy blocks the observed effects [8]. Microbial reconstitution can be undertaken, either by employing fecal microbial transplantation or by using a more targeted approach with either a combination of microbes or a single strain of what is considered to be a beneficial organism [9].

Probiotics are defined as live microorganisms which, if taken in sufficient amounts, have a benefit on health [10]. Increasing evidence shows that probiotics can reduce the symptoms of IBS in both children and adults. A meta-analysis of 23 randomized controlled trials evaluating the effectiveness of various probiotic strains in adults with IBS showed that the microbes are more effective than placebo (relative risk reduction of IBS of 0.79; 95% confidence intervals: 0.70–0.89; number needed to treat just 7; 95% confidence interval: 4–13) [11]. However, which individual microbial species and strains are the most beneficial awaits further direct head-to-head comparative trials.

Probiotics as a Management Strategy for Infant Colic

As summarized in Table 2, a number of trials indicate that the probiotic *Lactobacillus reuteri* (strain DSM 17928) provided at a dose of 1×10^8 bacteria, delivered as 5 drops once daily in a hydroscopic oil suspension for 3–4 weeks, is more effective than placebo in alleviating symptoms of fussiness and irritability in babies with colic [12]. Outcome measures include duration of infant crying and at least a 50% reduction in crying time versus baseline measures [13]. These prospective clinical studies were undertaken in Italy [14, 15], Poland [16], Australia [17], China [18], and Canada [19]. Another study conducted in Italy evaluated the effects of *L. reuteri* (strain DSM 17938) versus placebo over the first 90 days of life. At 3 months, crying time was significantly reduced in colicky babies receiving the probiotic (38 min/day) compared to infants randomized to the placebo arm of the study (71 min, $p < 0.01$). Moreover, there was a reduction in financial costs incurred for the families of infants with colic who received the probiotic agent [20]. A meta-analysis of the trials indicated that the active agent was more effective that placebo, with 5 of the 6 studies included in the evaluation having an impact that reached statistical significance [12]. A possible explanation for the negative trial undertaken in Australia could relate to a lower rate of exclusive breastfeeding compared to other studies. It should be noted that even though the total number of babies entered into all of the clinical trials is relatively small, there have been no serious adverse events reported.

How Might Probiotics Relieve Symptoms?

The underlying mechanism(s) that account for colic remain poorly understood. Nevertheless, as summarized in Figure 2, a compelling body of literature emphasizes that there is an active, dynamic, and bidirectional communication between the trillions of microbes colonizing the lumen and the mucous layer of the gut, with epithelial cells lining the intestine, and the underlying mucosal immune system and both the peripheral enteric and central nervous systems [21]. This has been termed the diet-microbiome-gut-brain axis. Recent evidence indicates that lactic acid-producing bacteria capable of catabolizing dietary tryptophan into a variety of indole derivatives mediate anti-inflammatory effects, both in the gut and in the central nervous system, via activation of the aryl hydrocarbon receptor and increased production of interleukin-22 by gut mucosa-resident T immune cells [22]. An accompanying editorial suggests that *L. reuteri* might be an effective probiotic choice to enhance the pathway of tryptophan metabolism as a novel anti-inflammatory strategy [23]. An additional mechanism that might be considered is that in an animal model of intestinal injury early in life, *L. reuteri* DSM 17938 increases the number of anti-inflammatory Foxp3+ regulatory T cells present in the intestinal mucosa [24].

Another potential consideration is that certain probiotic strains have a direct effect on visceral sensation. For instance, Perez-Burgoz et al. [25] reported that the firing frequency of the pronociceptive TRPV (transient receptor potential vanilloid) 1 channel in mesenteric spinal afferent nerve bundles in response to either small bowel luminal distension or capsaicin is reduced in the presence of bacterial cell-free culture supernatants derived from *L. reuteri* DSM 17928.

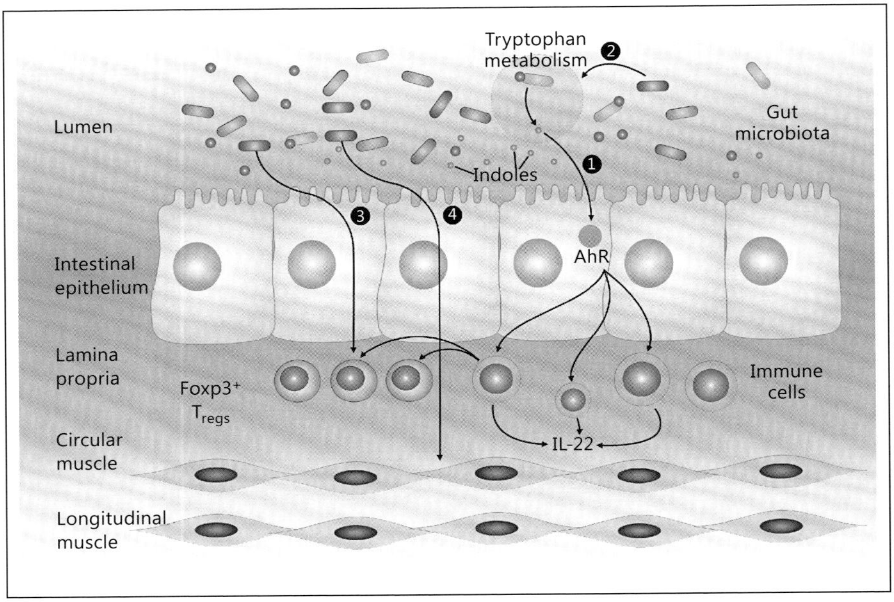

Fig. 2. Postulated mechanisms of action for probiotic-mediated benefits in infant colic. Lactic-acid bacteria metabolize tryptophan within the gastrointestinal tract into indole-derived molecules, which can bind aryl hydrocarbon receptors (AhR) to stimulate interleukin (IL)-22 production by T cells (1). Certain probiotic species, such as *Lactobacillus reuteri,* promote this process and thereby dampen mucosal inflammation (2). *L. reuteri* increases Foxp3+ regulatory T cells (T_{regs}) in the intestine, which has anti-inflammatory effects (3). *L. reuteri* DSM 17938 modulates smooth muscle contractions to regulate gut motility and promote intestinal transit (4).

Interestingly, the observed effects are strain specific with culture supernatants prepared from other lactic acid-producing bacteria having no antinociceptive effects. Alternatively, *L. reuteri* DSM 17928 may reduce symptoms of colic by mediating effects on gut motility and intestinal transit times [26]. Another possibility to consider as a potential underlying mechanism of action is provided by recent evidence showing that probiotics colonizing the gut of both rodents [27] and humans [28] can have a direct effect on the activity of neurotransmitters in the central nervous system.

Conclusions

Level 1 evidence secured from a number of prospective randomized controlled clinical trials shows that irritability in breastfed infants with colic can be better managed with probiotics than sham intervention alone. Issues related to the definition of entry criteria (that is, how best to define colic in a reproducible manner across centers and between studies) and measures employed as measures of primary outcome have appropriately been raised as issues of concern that warrant attention [29]. Nevertheless, the body of evidence accumulated to date and summarized in this review appears quite convincing. The studies have been undertaken in various countries in Europe, Asia, and North America with trials employing a single probiotic strain from the same commercial source. Dose escalation studies and head-to-head comparisons with other widely available probiotic strains and mixtures of strains in breastfed and formula-fed infants are now warranted [30]. Whether such an intervention early during the course of the life span will change the short- and long-term composition of the gut microbiome, mucosal immune function, and sensations of visceral pain requires ongoing study and continued surveillance of those subjects already entered into these clinical trials.

Acknowledgments

Work in the authors' laboratories is supported by the Swedish Society for Medical Research (to T.R.A.) and the Canadian Institutes of Health Research (CIHR; to P.M.S.). R.Y.W. is the recipient of a Vanier Graduate Scholarship Award from the CIHR, and P.M.S. is the recipient of a Canada Research Chair in Gastrointestinal Disease.

Disclosure Statement

T.R.A. has received honoraria for lectures and funding for a clinical trial from Biogaia AB, Sweden. P.M.S. has received honoraria from Abbott Nutrition, Mead Johnson Nutritionals and Nestlé Nutrition, and research supports from Lallemand Health Solutions.

References

1 Benninga MA, Nurko S, Faure C, et al: Childhood functional gastrointestinal disorders: neonate/toddler. Gastroenterology 2016;150:143–155.

2 Rajlic-Stojanovic M, Biagi E, Heilig HGHJ, et al: Global and deep molecular analysis of microbiota signatures in fecal samples from patients with irritable bowel syndrome. Gastroenterology 2011;141:1792–1801.

3 Saulnier DM, Riehle K, Mistretta T-A, et al: Gastrointestinal microbiome signatures of pediatric patients with irritable bowel syndrome. Gastroenterology 2011;141:1782–1791.

4 Cenac N, Andrews CN, Holzhuasen M, et al: Role for protease activity in visceral pain in irritable bowel syndrome. J Clin Invest 2007;117:636–647.

5 deWeerth C, Fuentes S, Puylaert P, et al: Intestinal microbiota of infants with colic: development and specific signatures. Pediatrics 2013;131:e550–e558.
6 Bauer KC, Huus KE, Finlay BB: Microbes and the mind: emerging hallmarks of the gut microbiota-brain axis. Cell Microbiol 2016;18: 632–644.
7 O'Mahony SM, Felice VD, Nally K, et al: Disturbance of the gut microbiota in early-life selectively affects visceral pain in adulthood without impacting cognitive or anxiety-related behaviors in male rats. Neuroscience 2014; 277:885–901.
8 Forsythe P, Bienenstock J, Kunze WA: Vagal pathways for microbiome-brain-gut axis communication. Adv Exp Biol 2014;817:115–133.
9 Buffie CG, Bucci V, Stein RR, et al: Precision microbiome reconstitution restores bile acid mediated resistance to *Clostridium difficile*. Nature 2015;517:205–208.
10 Hill C, Guarner F, Reid G, et al: The international Association for Probiotics and Prebiotics consensus statement on the scope and appropriate use of the term probiotic. Nat Rev Gastroenterol Hepatol 2014;11:506–514.
11 Ford AC, Quigley EMM, Lacy BE, et al: Efficacy of prebiotics, probiotics, and synbiotics in irritable bowel syndrome and chronic idiopathic constipation: systematic review and meta-analysis. Am J Gastroenterol 2014;109: 1547–1561.
12 Harb T, Matsuyama M, David M, et al: Infant colic – what works: a systematic review of interventions for breast-fed infants. J Pediatr Gastroenterol Nutr 2016;22:668–686.
13 Sung V, Cabana MD, D'Amico F, et al: *Lactobacillus reuteri* DSM 17938 for managing infant colic: protocol for an individual participant data meta-analysis. BMJ Open 2014; 4:e006475.
14 Savino F, Pelle E, Palumeri E, et al: *Lactobacillus reuteri* (American Type Culture Collection strain 55730) versus simethicone in the treatment of infantile colic: a prospective randomized study. Pediatrics 2007;119:e124–e130.
15 Savino F, Cordisco L, Tarasco V, et al: *Lactobacillus reuteri* DSM 17938 in infantile colic: a randomized, double-blind, placebo-controlled trial. Pediatrics 2010;126:e526–e533.
16 Szajewska H, Gyrczuk E, Horvath A: *Lactobacillus reuteri* DSM 17938 for the management of infantile colic in breastfed infants: a randomized, double-blind, placebo-controlled trial. J Pediatr 2013;162:257–262.
17 Sung V, Hiscock H, Tang MLK, et al: Treating infant colic with the probiotic *Lactobacillus reuteri*: double blind, placebo controlled randomised trial. Br Med J 2014;348:g2107.
18 Mi GL, Zhao L, Qiao DD, et al: Effectiveness of *Lactobacillus reuteri* in infantile colic and colicky induced maternal depression: a prospective single blind randomized trial. Antonie Van Leeuwenhoek 2015;107:1547–1553.
19 Chau K, Lau E, Greenberg S, et al: Probiotics for infantile colic: a randomized, double-blind, placebo-controlled trial investigating *Lactobacillus reuteri* DSM 17938. J Pediatr 2015;166:74–78.
20 Indrio F, DiMauro A, Riezzo G, et al: Prophylactic use of a probiotic in the prevention of colic, regurgitation, and functional constipation. A randomized clinical trial. JAMA Pediatr 2014;168:228–233.
21 Hsiao EY, McBride SW, Hsien S, et al: Microbiota modulate behavioural and physiological abnormalities associated with neurodevelopmental disorders. Cell 2013;155:1–13.
22 Lamas B, Richard ML, Deducq V, et al: CARD9 impacts colitis by altering gut microbiota metabolism of tryptophan into aryl hydrocarbon receptors. Nat Med 2016;22:598–605.
23 Marsland BJ: Regulating inflammation with microbial metabolites. Nat Med 2016;22:581–583.
24 Liu Y, Tran DQ, Fatheree NY, et al: *Lactobacillus reuteri* DSM 17938 differentially modulates effector memory T cells and Foxp3+ regulatory T cell in a mouse model of necrotizing enterocolitis. Am J Physiol 2014; 307:G177–G186.
25 Perez-Burgos A, Wang L, McVey Neufeld K-A, et al: The TRPV1 channel in rodents is a major target for antinociceptive effect of the probiotic *Lactobacillus reuteri* DSM 17938. J Physiol 2015;593:3943–3957.
26 Wu RY, Pasyk M, Wang B, et al: Spatiotemporal maps reveal regional differences in the effects on gut motility for *Lactobacillus reuteri* and *L. rhamnosus* strains. Neurogastroenterol Motil 2013;25:e205–e214.

27 Janik R, Thomason JAM, Stanisz AM, et al: Magnetic resonance spectroscopy reveals oral *Lactobacillus* promotion of increases in brain GABA, N-acetyl aspartate and glutamate. NeuroImage 2016;125:988–995.
28 Tillisch K, Labus J, Kilpatrick L, et al: Consumption of fermented milk products with probiotic modulates brain activity. Gastroenterology 2013;144:1394–1401.
29 Steutel NF, Benninga MA, Langendam MW, et al: Reporting outcome measures in trials of infant colic. J Pediatr Gastroenterol Nutr 2014;59:341–346.
30 Abrahamsson T, Rautava S, Moore A, et al: The time for a confirmative necrotizing enterocolitis probiotics prevention trial in the extremely low birth weight infant in North America is now! J Pediatr 2014;165:389–394.

Isolauri E, Sherman PM, Walker WA (eds): Intestinal Microbiome: Functional Aspects in Health and Disease. Nestlé Nutr Inst Workshop Ser, vol 88, pp 117–126, (DOI: 10.1159/000455220)
Nestec Ltd., Vevey/S. Karger AG., Basel, © 2017

Diet and Gut Microbiota in Health and Disease

Ting-Chin David Shen

Division of Gastroenterology, Perelman School of Medicine, University of Pennsylvania, Philadelphia, PA, USA

Abstract

Gut microbiota plays an important role in host health maintenance and disease pathogenesis. The development of a stable and diverse gut microbiota is essential to various host physiologic functions such as immunoregulation, pathogen prevention, energy harvest, and metabolism. At the same time, a dysbiotic gut microbiota associated with disease is altered in structure and function, and often characterized by a decrease in species richness and proliferation of pathogenic bacterial taxa. As a shared substrate between the host and the gut microbiota, diet significantly impacts the health and disease states of the host both directly and through gut microbial metabolite production. This is demonstrated in the examples of short-chain fatty acid and trimethylamine production via bacterial metabolism of dietary complex carbohydrates and choline, respectively. In disorders related to mucosal immune dysregulation such as inflammatory bowel disease, the dysbiotic gut microbiota and diet contribute to its pathogenesis. Reversal of dysbiosis through fecal microbiota transplantation and dietary interventions may thus represent important strategies to modify the gut microbiota and its metabolite production for health maintenance as well as disease prevention and management.

Introduction

We coexist with trillions of microorganisms that reside on our various mucosal surfaces, including the skin and respiratory, genitourinary, and gastrointestinal (GI) tracts. These microorganisms comprise bacteria, fungi, viruses, and archaea, and are collectively known as our microbiota. They have evolved with our body to help us to maintain health in various ways such as immunoregulation, pathogen prevention, energy harvest, and metabolism [1, 2]. At the same time, the microbiota can become altered in structure and function by host and/or environmental factors. In the setting of disease, this is known as dysbiosis. Dysbiosis has been associated with various diseases, including diabetes, atherosclerosis, asthma, cancer, and inflammatory bowel disease (IBD) [3]. In this review, we will focus on the microbiota that inhabits our GI tract, otherwise known as the gut microbiota, and its interactions with diet. We will examine how the intricate and dynamic interplay between diet and gut microbiota affects both the health and disease states of the host.

Early Gut Microbiota Development

From birth, we are exposed to various microorganisms in our environment that gradually colonize our GI tract and become part of our gut microbiota. Various substances enter the body through the mouth and interact with the gut microbiota. These include food, antibiotics, and xenobiotics, each of which can exert strong and direct effects on the body and the gut microbiota, which in turn mediate downstream effects on the host. For example, the use of antibiotics can deplete certain endogenous microbial populations within the GI tract, allowing opportunistic pathogens to proliferate, as in the case of *Clostridium difficile* infection [4]. This infection results in severe diarrhea and abdominal pain that is frequently relapsing and refractory to conventional medical treatment. The use of fecal microbiota transplantation (FMT) from healthy donors has been shown to dramatically induce remission and prevent relapse [5]. The use of antibiotics early in life has also been linked to the development of obesity [6]. One study showed that low-dose antibiotic treatment (i.e. penicillin) of preweaning murine pups led to increased and lasting adiposity [7]. The metabolic consequences are likely secondary to altered gut microbiota rather than the effects of the antibiotic itself, as the obese phenotype is transferred to germ-free mice that received FMT from antibiotic-treated mice but not from control mice. These findings point to the critical time in infancy during which changes that affect either the host or the gut microbiota can have lasting metabolic effects on the other. For example, the cessation of breastfeeding correlates with the transition of microbiota to a more "adult-like" microbiome state with increased diversity and stability that may be critical for health with long-term consequences on growth and development. One recent study found that Malawian mothers with stunted infants have decreased levels of sialylated milk oligosaccharides compared to those with healthy infants [8]. Furthermore, the transfer of fecal microbiota from a stunted Malawian infant to gnotobiotic mice and piglets led to improved growth on a Malawian diet supplemented with sialylated milk oligosaccharides compared to a diet without sialylated milk oligosaccharides.

Diet and Gut Microbiota

The gut microbiota interacts with diet to affect host physiology and metabolism. Differences in the composition of the gut microbiota among individuals may explain the interindividual variations in response to the same dietary modifications. In a recent study, investigators compared the microbiota of participants that demonstrated improved glucose metabolism after administration of a short-term supplementation of barley kernel-based bread to those that did not respond [9]. They found a higher *Prevotella/Bacteroides* ratio in the responders, consistent with metagenomic analysis results showing an increased potential to ferment complex carbohydrates. This supports a personalized approach to improve metabolism based on analyses of gut microbial composition and function as well as dietary interventions. Another study found that there is high variability in postprandial glycemic response (PPGR) among an 800-person cohort after consuming standardized meals [10]. By collecting clinical and microbiota metagenomic data and integrating them into an algorithm, the investigators were able to accurately predict PPGR in a second independent cohort as well as personalize dietary interventions to reduce PPGR with consistent changes in gut microbiota composition. Other studies have quantified and accurately predicted fecal and blood metabolomics data using mathematical modeling of the human gut microbiome and its interactions with diet and the host [11].

The typical high-fat, high-sugar "Western" diet has been associated with decreases in gut microbial diversity, whereas an agrarian diet, rich in fruits and vegetables with high fiber content, is associated with increased bacterial gene richness [12]. Diet may affect the composition of the gut microbiota, although the extent of this effect remains controversial. Prior studies have suggested that different human populations may be grouped into distinct clusters based on the predominant bacterial taxa associated with different dietary patterns. For example, agrarian-based cultures that consume a plant-based diet generally have higher relative abundance of *Prevotella*, whereas industrialized populations that consume more animal proteins and fats generally have higher relative abundance of *Bacteroides* [12]. Other studies have demonstrated that the impact of diet on the gut microbiota composition may be less prominent. In a study that examined the gut microbiota of omnivores and vegans residing in an urban environment in the United States, differences in the gut microbiota between both

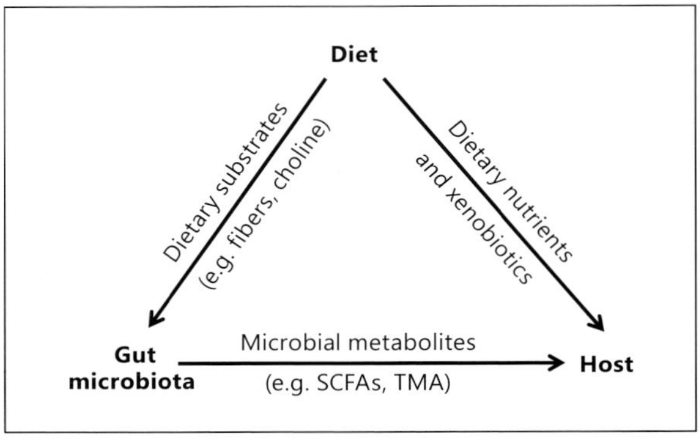

Fig. 1. Interactions among diet, the gut microbiota, and the host. Diet is a substrate shared by the gut microbiota and the host, affecting host health and disease both through direct absorption of dietary components and microbial metabolite production. SCFAs, short chain fatty acids; TMA, trimethylamine.

cohorts were surprisingly small [13]. Nevertheless, the plasma metabolomes of omnivores and vegans differed significantly, with omnivores having more amino acid and lipid metabolites from the consumption of animal products, and vegans having more metabolites from plant-based products via bacterial metabolism. Overall, a significant shift in the structure of the gut microbiota may reflect long-term dietary changes and/or additional environmental influences [13, 14].

Diet and Microbial Metabolites

As a shared substrate between the host and the gut microbiota, diet affects the host via both direct intestinal absorption and microbial metabolite production with downstream effects (Fig. 1). One prime example is the fermentation of dietary complex carbohydrates by gut microbiota to produce short-chain fatty acids (SCFAs) such as acetate, butyrate, and propionate. Certain bacterial species, including *Bacteroides thetaiotaomicron* and *B. ovatus*, contain more glycosidases and lyases than humans and thereby are able to metabolize nearly all the glycans in dietary fibers [2]. SCFAs perform a variety of functions. Butyrate serves as an important energy substrate for the colonic epithelium, where it can also affect proliferation, differentiation, and modulation of gene expression by inhibiting histone deacetylase [2]. Acetate and propionate can reach various organs through the bloodstream and serve as substrates for lipogenesis and gluconeogenesis as well as regulate different gene expressions by binding to G protein-coupled receptors GPR41 and GPR43 [1]. The end-organ effects of SCFAs through these receptors depend on the cell type. For example, SCFAs can modulate secretion of the hormone glucagon-like peptide-1 (GLP-1) through effects on enteroendocrine L cells in the distal small intestine and colon, thereby improving insulin secretion [1]. On the other hand, SCFAs suppress inflammation in neutrophils via GPR43 signaling. SCFAs have also been shown to play a role in mucosal immune tolerance through regulation of colonic regulatory T cells [15].

Risk of Cardiovascular Disease

Another dietary component that strongly impacts upon the health of the host via gut microbial metabolism is choline. Choline is predominantly obtained from the diet in foods such as red meat and eggs, although it can also be synthesized by the host [2]. Choline is primarily metabolized in the liver, where it plays a role in lipid metabolism and the synthesis of very-low-density lipoprotein. The gut microbiota can also metabolize dietary choline to produce trimethylamine (TMA) through the enzymatic activity of choline TMA-lyase, which is encoded by the CutC gene carried by both human commensal and pathogenic bacteria [16]. TMA is further metabolized in the liver by the flavin monooxygenase system to produce TMA-N-oxide (TMAO), which has shown to be associated with the development of atherosclerosis and cardiovascular diseases [17]. Strategies to reduce the risk of cardiovascular disease from dietary choline consumption and microbial TMA production include interventions that reduce the representation of CutC-expressing gut bacteria and/or inhibit microbial TMA-lyase activity. As proof of concept, one study demonstrated that a structural analog of choline, 3,3-dimethyl-1-butanol (DMB), can nonlethally inhibit microbial TMA-lyase and TMA production to reduce TMAO levels in mice fed a high-choline diet [18]. DMB further inhibited choline diet-enhanced endogenous macrophage foam cell formation and atherosclerotic lesion development in mice. By compiling clinical, metagenomic, and metabolomic data, one can develop a comprehensive and individualized plan to not only prognosticate the risk of cardiovascular disease in association with choline consumption and gut microbial TMA production, but also prevent and manage disease risk via modulation of the gut microbiota.

Effect of Chronic Kidney Disease

Microbial metabolites such as TMA cross the intestinal epithelium to enter the body and circulate in the plasma. A steady state of the microbial metabolites in the host is then determined by a balance between input (from dietary substrate intake and subsequent microbial metabolism) and output (primarily via renal excretion). Changes in either can alter the plasma metabolome equilibrium. Patients with chronic kidney disease and decreased glomerular filtration rate may not be able to properly and efficiently excrete toxic metabolites that can lead to disease. Indeed, it has been shown that the age-adjusted risks of death and cardiovascular events vary inversely with the estimated glomerular filtration rate [19]. Also, TMA and TMAO levels were found to be elevated in patients with

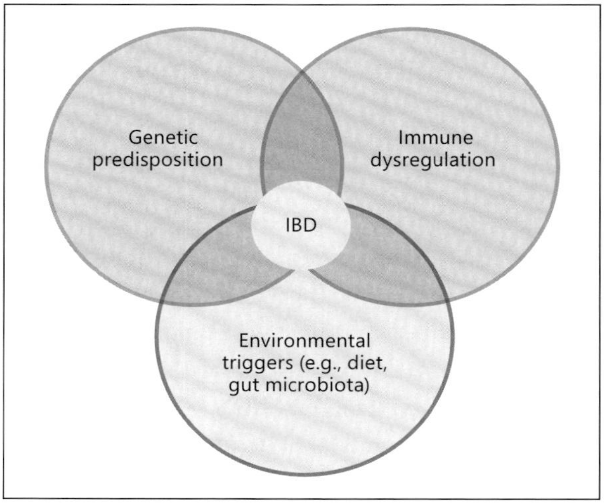

Fig. 2. Pathogenesis of IBD. In genetically predisposed individuals, mucosal immune dysregulation and environmental triggers such as diet and the gut microbiota elicit severe host inflammatory responses and lead to symptoms.

end-stage renal disease [20]. These findings suggest that the determination of renal excretion of microbial metabolites may be important in cardiovascular disease prevention and management. Researcher who examine and characterize the abundance of additional metabolites that vary between healthy subjects and chronic kidney disease patients may reveal novel associations between microbial metabolites and host metabolic pathways linked to disease.

Inflammatory Bowel Disease

In addition to its role in cardiovascular disease, the gut microbiota impacts the development of inflammatory bowel disease (IBD). IBD represents a group of inflammatory disorders that primarily affect the GI tract, and Crohn disease (CD) and ulcerative colitis (UC) are the two most common types. CD presents with ulcerations anywhere along the GI tract from the mouth to the anus, whereas UC is restricted to the colon, but both can have extraintestinal manifestations that involve the skin, joints, and eyes. Over the past few decades, the incidence of IBD has risen globally [21], which may be related to improved diagnosis rates but also to potential changes to our diet and/or gut microbiota. The pathogenesis of IBD is multifactorial and incompletely elucidated. Genetic predisposition, immune system dysregulation, and environmental triggers all play a role (Fig. 2). The genetic contribution to the development of CD is found to be at most 30–40%, where the total contribution of all 163 IBD-associated genetic loci account for only 13% of CD variance [22]. This suggests that environmental factors likely represent the greatest contributor to the pathogenesis of IBD.

Current approaches to IBD treatment focus primarily on immunosuppression through medications such as biologics, immunomodulators, and corticosteroids. These therapies reduce intestinal inflammation without modifying its triggers, which may be related to luminal antigens in the diet and/or gut microbiota but remain incompletely characterized. At the same time, intestinal inflammation contributes to a dysbiotic microbiota in IBD, marked by a decrease in species richness as well as the proliferation of certain pathogenic bacterial taxa [22]. Studies have shown that the abundance of Bacteroidetes and Firmicutes, two dominant phyla in the human gut microbiota, decrease in IBD, whereas Proteobacteria such as Enterobacteriaceae increase in abundance. However, it is unclear if intestinal inflammation and changes in the redox potential of the intestinal milieu lead to the development of a dysbiotic microbiota with increased facultative anaerobes, or whether dysbiosis promotes the persistence of intestinal inflammation [23].

Fecal Microbiota Transplantation

Reversing dysbiosis through FMT represents a novel approach to IBD treatment. Two randomized clinical trials have investigated the use of FMT in UC with conflicting results. Moayyedi et al. [24] performed FMT via enema using stool from healthy unrelated donors given weekly for 6 weeks and found significantly higher remission rates at week 7 compared to the use of water enema as placebo (24 vs. 5%; $p = 0.03$). Subgroup analyses revealed that the efficacy of FMT in UC may be donor dependent, and remission rates may be higher if FMT is performed early in the disease course. On the other hand, Rossen et al. [25] found that UC patients who received FMT by nasoduodenal tube at weeks 0 and 3 using stool from healthy donors showed no difference in remission rates at week 12 compared to those that received autologous FMT as placebo (30.4 vs. 20%; $p = 0.51$). The major differences between both studies include the route and frequency of FMT administration. In the case of CD, no randomized clinical trials have been completed to date, although 4 case series involving 38 patients with CD showed a clinical response to FMT in 60.5% (95% CI 28–86%) [26]. In short, additional large-scale randomized controlled studies are needed before FMT can be recommended as a therapy for IBD.

Exclusive Enteral Nutrition

The use of defined formula diets has been investigated extensively for the treatment of IBD, in particular CD. Numerous studies in IBD patients as well as in murine models of colitis have shown that exclusive enteral nutrition (EEN), whether it is elemental, semi-elemental, or polymeric, can induce remission in CD and promote mucosal healing. In particular, one study demonstrated that EEN was as effective in inducing clinical remission and more effective than corticosteroids in mucosal healing [27], potentially sparing the adverse effects of corticosteroids on the development of and bone growth in children. However, studies have demonstrated less efficacy of EEN in treating UC or CD primarily involving the colon. Interestingly, the efficacy of EEN may not be dependent on the composition of the formula. A Cochrane review found no significant difference in efficacy among different formulations of EEN based on protein or fat content [28]. The exact mechanisms by which EEN ameliorates CD remain unclear and may include improved nutrition, exclusion or reduction in luminal antigens derived from food, direct anti-inflammatory effects of the formula, or changes in the gut microbiota [22]. Indeed, it is possible that EEN may eliminate some harmful substances in processed foods, as 2 recent studies showed that artificial sweeteners and dietary emulsifiers can affect the gut microbiota leading to metabolic disturbances and inflammation [29, 30].

Conclusion

In conclusion, both our gut microbiota and diet can strongly impact our health, with the effects of one mediated by the availability and property of the other. Dietary substrates can have beneficial and/or adverse effects on our body through direct absorption across the intestinal epithelium upon food passage through the GI tract. At the same time, the effects of various dietary components may not be fully realized without the metabolic capacity of the gut microbiota. The development of a rich and stable gut microbiota is crucial for the proper development of many host physiologic functions. In the setting of disease, the dysbiotic gut microbiota is characterized by decreased diversity and the predominance of a few pathogenic taxa which can adversely affect host health. Gut microbiota affects host health primarily through the metabolites they produce, which is strongly dependent upon the substrates available through dietary intake. Furthermore, diet can shape both the structure and the function of gut microbiota. The future of gut microbial medicine lies in an individualized approach based on a comprehensive analysis of the unique gut microbiomes different individuals possess and their dietary intake, taking into account their genetic and epigenetic predispositions. A better understanding of the intricate and dynamic relationship between diet, the gut microbiota, and the host is crucial for enhancing health and preventing disease.

Disclosure Statement

Conflict of interest: none.

References

1 Nicholson JK, Holmes E, Kinross J, et al: Host-gut microbiota metabolic interactions. Science 2012;336:1262–1267.

2 Tremaroli V, Backhed F: Functional interactions between the gut microbiota and host metabolism. Nature 2012;489:242–249.

3 Sommer F, Backhed F: The gut microbiota – masters of host development and physiology. Nat Rev Microbiol 2013;11:227–238.

4 Rupnik M, Wilcox MH, Gerding DN: Clostridium difficile infection: new developments in epidemiology and pathogenesis. Nat Rev Microbiol 2009;7:526–536.

5 Petrof EO, Khoruts A: From stool transplants to next-generation microbiota therapeutics. Gastroenterology 2014;146:1573–1582.

6 Cho I, Yamanishi S, Cox L, et al: Antibiotics in early life alter the murine colonic microbiome and adiposity. Nature 2012;488:621–626.

7 Cox LM, Yamanishi S, Sohn J, et al: Altering the intestinal microbiota during a critical developmental window has lasting metabolic consequences. Cell 2014;158:705–721.

8 Charbonneau MR, O'Donnell D, Blanton LV, et al: Sialylated milk oligosaccharides promote microbiota-dependent growth in models of infant undernutrition. Cell 2016;164: 859–871.

9 Kovatcheva-Datchary P, Nilsson A, Akrami R, et al: Dietary fiber-induced improvement in glucose metabolism is associated with increased abundance of Prevotella. Cell Metab 2015;22:971–982.

10 Zeevi D, Korem T, Zmora N, et al: Personalized nutrition by prediction of glycemic responses. Cell 2015;163:1079–1094.

11 Shoaie S, Ghaffari P, Kovatcheva-Datchary P, et al: Quantifying diet-induced metabolic changes of the human gut microbiome. Cell Metab 2015;22:320–331.

12 De Filippo C, Cavalieri D, Di Paola M, et al: Impact of diet in shaping gut microbiota revealed by a comparative study in children from Europe and rural Africa. Proc Natl Acad Sci U S A 2010;107:14691–14696.

13 Wu GD, Compher C, Chen EZ, et al: Comparative metabolomics in vegans and omnivores reveal constraints on diet-dependent gut microbiota metabolite production. Gut 2016;65:63–72.

14 Wu GD, Chen J, Hoffmann C, et al: Linking long-term dietary patterns with gut microbial enterotypes. Science 2011;334:105–108.

15 Smith PM, Howitt MR, Panikov N, et al: The microbial metabolites, short-chain fatty acids, regulate colonic Treg cell homeostasis. Science 2013;341:569–573.

16 Craciun S, Balskus EP: Microbial conversion of choline to trimethylamine requires a glycyl radical enzyme. Proc Natl Acad Sci U S A 2012;109:21307–21312.

17 Wang Z, Klipfell E, Bennett BJ, et al: Gut flora metabolism of phosphatidylcholine promotes cardiovascular disease. Nature 2011; 472:57–63.

18 Wang Z, Roberts AB, Buffa JA, et al: Nonlethal inhibition of gut microbial trimethylamine production for the treatment of atherosclerosis. Cell 2015;163:1585–1595.

19 Go AS, Chertow GM, Fan D, et al: Chronic kidney disease and the risks of death, cardiovascular events, and hospitalization. N Engl J Med 2004;351:1296–1305.

20 Bain MA, Faull R, Fornasini G, et al: Accumulation of trimethylamine and trimethylamine-N-oxide in end-stage renal disease patients undergoing haemodialysis. Nephrol Dial Transplant 2006;21:1300–1304.

21 Molodecky NA, Soon IS, Rabi DM, et al: Increasing incidence and prevalence of the inflammatory bowel diseases with time, based on systematic review. Gastroenterology 2012; 142:46–54.e42; quiz e30.

22 Lee D, Albenberg L, Compher C, et al: Diet in the pathogenesis and treatment of inflammatory bowel diseases. Gastroenterology 2015; 148:1087–1106.

23 Sartor RB: Therapeutic correction of bacterial dysbiosis discovered by molecular techniques. Proc Natl Acad Sci U S A 2008;105: 16413–16414.

24 Moayyedi P, Surette MG, Kim PT, et al: Fecal microbiota transplantation induces remission in patients with active ulcerative colitis in a randomized controlled trial. Gastroenterology 2015;149:102–109.e6.

25 Rossen NG, Fuentes S, van der Spek MJ, et al: Findings from a randomized controlled trial of fecal transplantation for patients with ulcerative colitis. Gastroenterology 2015;149: 110–118.e4.

26 Colman RJ, Rubin DT: Fecal microbiota transplantation as therapy for inflammatory bowel disease: a systematic review and meta-analysis. J Crohns Colitis 2014;8:1569–1581.
27 Borrelli O, Cordischi L, Cirulli M, et al: Polymeric diet alone versus corticosteroids in the treatment of active pediatric Crohn's disease: a randomized controlled open-label trial. Clin Gastroenterol Hepatol 2006;4:744–753.
28 Zachos M, Tondeur M, Griffiths AM: Enteral nutritional therapy for induction of remission in Crohn's disease. Cochrane Database Syst Rev 2007;1:CD000542.
29 Suez J, Korem T, Zeevi D, et al: Artificial sweeteners induce glucose intolerance by altering the gut microbiota. Nature 2014;514:181–186.
30 Chassaing B, Koren O, Goodrich JK, et al: Dietary emulsifiers impact the mouse gut microbiota promoting colitis and metabolic syndrome. Nature 2015;519:92–96.

Isolauri E, Sherman PM, Walker WA (eds): Intestinal Microbiome: Functional Aspects in Health and Disease. Nestlé Nutr Inst Workshop Ser, vol 88, pp 127–128, (DOI: 10.1159/000455221)
Nestec Ltd., Vevey/S. Karger AG., Basel, © 2017

Summary of Normal Development of Gut Microbiota and Dysbiosis

Session II set the stage for understanding the clinical correlates and consequences of dysbiosis. Dysbiosis indicates a shift in gut microbiota composition, i.e., an imbalance in the taxonomic composition appropriate for the age and the environment of the host. Critical evaluation was made of early-life exposures and clinical practices, which may interfere with the normal compositional development of gut microbiota and thereby carry a risk of future disease.

Josef Neu discussed dysbiosis in the neonatal period focusing on the mode of delivery. In point of fact, the rate of cesarean section delivery exceeds the WHO recommendation in most parts of the world. He underlined the importance of this critical period of maturation; early-life perturbations of the microbiota, dysbioses, are likely to lead to metabolic, immunologic, and epigenetic consequences, and perhaps may even effect subsequent generations. Children born by cesarean section have an increased susceptibility to several immune-related conditions including asthma, type I diabetes, food allergies, allergic rhinitis, and celiac disease.

Sanjay Patole reviewed the evidence that gut microbiota composition in infants born preterm creates the risk of necrotizing enterocolitis (NEC). NEC is an acquired inflammatory condition of the gut and a common cause of mortality and morbidity in preterm infants with very low birth weight. The early postnatal gut microbiota of preterm infants is typified as simple, very diverse, and dynamic, thereby an important determinant in the development of NEC. However, the possibility that changes in gut microbiota may be a consequence rather than a cause of NEC in preterm infants calls for further research in this area.

Meghan B. Azad and colleagues studied the impact of early-life antibiotic exposure on the risk of obesity later in life. Cesarean section delivery is regularly accompanied by antibiotic use. Both clinical and experimental evidence indicates that antibiotic exposure during critical periods of early development may disrupt the normal colonization, alter the "programming" of weight gain trajectories, and lead to the development of obesity.

Erika Isolauri presented epidemiological, experimental, and clinical data pointing to a causative role of the gut microbiota in obesity. In addition to processing nutrients and regulating their access to and storage in the body, activated inflammatory pathways are a corollary to "obesogenic microbiota". A distinctive gut microbiota composition prevails in obese individuals, with adjustments following weight gain or weight loss. Thus, modification of gut microbial communities might offer a strategy to manage obesity.

Philip M. Sherman and colleagues revised the etiologic role of dysbiosis in functional gastrointestinal disorders: colic in infants and irritable bowel syndrome (IBD) in older children and adults. Reduced diversity and low numbers of bifidobacteria and lactobacilli have been detected in infants who went on to develop colic, and modification of gut microbiota by specific probiotics alleviates the condition. Whether such interventions early in life will provide long-term clinical benefit requires continued surveillance of those subjects already entered into clinical trials.

Ting-Chin David Shen evaluated the interaction of diet and microbiota in health and disease. He underlined that diet impacts on the health of the host not only through a direct nutritional effect but also via the gut microbiota through microbial metabolite production. Butyrate, for example, serves as an important energy substrate for the colonic epithelium, while acetate and propionate act as substrates for lipogenesis and gluconeogenesis, and regulate different gene expression. These are particularly relevant in chronic inflammatory conditions such as IBD. However, it remains to be elucidated if intestinal inflammation leads to the development of dysbiosis or dysbiosis perpetuates intestinal inflammation. Nevertheless, modulation of the gut microbiota is considered to represent an important strategy to treat IBD.

Erika Isolauri

Isolauri E, Sherman PM, Walker WA (eds): Intestinal Microbiome: Functional Aspects in Health and Disease. Nestlé Nutr Inst Workshop Ser, vol 88, pp 129–136, (DOI: 10.1159/000455250)
Nestec Ltd., Vevey/S. Karger AG., Basel, © 2017

Enzymes in Human Milk

David C. Dallas[a] · J. Bruce German[b]

[a]Nutrition Program, School of Biological and Population Health Sciences, College of Public Health and Human Sciences, Oregon State University, Corvallis, OR, and [b]Foods for Health Institute, University of California, Davis, Davis, CA, USA

Abstract

Milk proteins are a complex and diverse source of biological activities. Beyond their function, intact milk proteins also act as carriers of encrypted functional sequences that, when released as peptides, exert biological functions, including antimicrobial and immunomodulatory activity, which could contribute to the infant's competitive success. Research has now revealed that the release of these functional peptides begins within the mammary gland itself. A complex array of proteases produced in mother's milk has been shown to be active in the milk, releasing these peptides. Moreover, our recent research demonstrates that these milk proteases continue to digest milk proteins within the infant's stomach, possibly even to a larger extent than the infant's own proteases. As the neonate has relatively low digestive capacity, the activity of milk proteases in the infant may provide important assistance to digesting milk proteins. The coordinated release of these encrypted sequences is accomplished by selective proteolytic action provided by an array of native milk proteases and infant-produced enzymes. The task for scientists is now to discover the selective advantages of this protein-protease-based peptide release system.

Introduction

As scientists have interrogated mammalian lactation and its remarkable product milk as a complete, comprehensive, and sustaining diet for mammalian infants, it has become increasingly clear that the simple term 'milk' does not do justice to this complex process. Using the term "milk" implies that there is such a thing as a single, ideal sample of this biofluid with a sole definable composition of nutrients. In fact, milk is highly dynamic, with many aspects changing constantly throughout the duration of lactation. Scientists must now develop research models that address this dynamic nature of milk. It is also as important to annotate the consequences of the changes in milk as well as the simple compositional diversity. Ultimately, the dynamic dimension of lactation must be understood in terms of its relevance to the nourishment of infants and the protection of the maternal investment. In addition to understanding the temporal dimension, milk is also biologically active, containing enzymes, antibodies, cells, and microorganisms. Unfortunately, this dimension too is poorly understood and the "proof" of this is the way milk is processed today. The vast majority of these biologically active components, structures, and organisms are irreversibly inactivated by the storage and stabilization processes that are applied to human milk if not consumed immediately and, of course, are unavailable in current generation infant formula.

The biological processes that constitute the full dimension of mammalian lactation evolved under the relentless pressure of darwinian evolution through the genetic success of the mother-infant pair. This evolutionary perspective of milk is considering the unique set of selective pressures that have shaped lactation over more than 200 million years [1]. Every milk component costs the mother. Without benefit to the infant, all components, especially those that are essential nutrients, are under negative selective pressure due to the cost to the mother's survival. Thus, while most research has focused on the nutritional value of milk to infants as a complete diet, lactation properties that supported acute protection of the maternal-infant dyad and the successful long-term development of the infant are also selectable traits. Research on the proteins of milk are beginning to reveal a more complex nutrition and protection system than previously considered, tailored to individual infants targeted to specific stages of development. Furthermore, proteins are emerging as a much more complex and diverse source of biological activities. Proteins as biopolymers possess distinct properties intact, which act also as carriers of encrypted functional sequences that when released as peptides add distinct properties. The coordinated release of these encrypted sequences is accomplished by selective proteolytic action provided by an array of native milk proteases and infant-produced enzymes. Now the task for scientists is to discover the selective advantages of this protein-protease-based peptide release system. The evidence to date suggests that these peptides have antimicrobial, immunomodulatory, and other functions that protect the infant from pathogens, guide development, and contribute in diverse ways to the infant's competitive success.

A New Model for Protein Nutrition

The current paradigm for protein nourishment in humans is that intact proteins are denatured by stomach acid and attacked by endogenous proteases in the stomach beginning a digestive process that continues with hydrolysis by neutral proteases in the small intestine ultimately leading to the release and complete absorption of amino acids by the intestinal epithelia. Young infants, however, are developmentally naïve, produce relatively little gastric acid, and express relatively low protease activity. Nonetheless, all evidence suggests that infants digest and absorb milk proteins effectively. How is this possible? The explanation for this apparent inconsistency comes from recent research showing that milk itself contains an array of proteases that are activated within the infant and contribute considerable catalytic activity and specificity to the entire process of protein digestion within the infant. This research is also revealing that in addition to aiding the infant in protein digestion per se, the specificity of digestion is so precise that there is in practice a further role for milk proteins: that they serve as carriers of encrypted peptide fragments that, upon release by selective proteases, exert functions that contribute to infant protection, health, and development.

A long and successful history of research has defined the intestinal enzymes capable of digesting proteins within the human gut. Studies have also been conducted on this repertoire of enzymes and their actions on milk proteins, and have identified a large number of peptides released from milk proteins [2, 3]. Parallel studies have examined the actions of milk peptides, including antimicrobial and anti-inflammatory functions, mucosal healing, blood pressure lowering, antithrombotic activity, and calcium delivery [4]. A new set of tools are emerging from chemistry, genomics, computational biology, and clinical medicine that are being directed to understanding digestion within the gastrointestinal tract of actual infants, to identifying the peptides that are actually present within breastfed infants, the enzymes responsible for releasing them, and the biological properties that they can potentially provide to preterm infants. This principle has been demonstrated using samples from full-term and premature infants with indwelling gastric feeding tubes combined with state-of-the-art analytics capable of determining peptide sequences with mass spectrometry and database searching and predict their functions with bioinformatic tools [5, 6].

The identification of hundreds of novel peptides was made possible by revolutionary breakthroughs in analytical chemistry of peptides [7]. Mapping these peptides to biological actions will be a major challenge for biologists as they seek to annotate their functional roles, including antimicrobial and immunomodulatory activities [3, 7]. These peptides have already been proposed to have a range of roles in protecting, nourishing and guiding the development of the infant and also protecting the mother from mammary infection.

This exciting research field that is continuing to reveal structures and functions of milk proteins provide insights into far more than how to nourish infants. The targets of action, mechanisms of health protection, and candidate ingredients are envisioned to assist with the support of premature infants whose enzyme repertoires are naive, the elderly whose digestive capacities are diminished, and clinical patients whose intestinal functions are pharmacologically impaired. There is a new optimism the lessons from milk's proteins and peptides will contribute to the health and development of people of all ages.

Research Discovery

The proteolysis of milk proteins was originally documented and perceived as a defect in individual milk samples. For example, the high protease activity in milk from cows with mastitis was associated with casein degradation and lower cheese yields [8]. This endogenous "defect" concept continued to dominate the scientific perspective of milk proteolysis in part because of the lack of tools to interrogate the degree of specificity of the process. The emergence of highly sensitive and accurate analytical tools capable of analyzing peptides is making it now possible to examine milk in much greater detail and quantitative accuracy [9]. These tools have been applied to examining human milk intact and as it is digested within the infant stomach [3, 5]. The first question that was asked was simple: are peptides released from human milk proteins within the infant intestine? The results (Fig. 1, 2) graphically document (1) that "native" milk, i.e. human milk samples prior to consumption by the infant, contain a diverse array of peptides and (2) that peptide diversity and abundance rise rapidly within the infant stomach.

Enzymatic Proteolysis of Milk

The specificity and reproducibility of the digestion of milk proteins provides convincing evidence of a complex, yet controlled, active proteolytic system. The origin of that proteolysis began to emerge from studies that showed that hydrolysis of specific milk proteins begins within the mammary gland itself [3]. Once reaching the stomach of the infant, proteolysis and release of peptides continues to show considerable protein selectivity and linkage specificity. It is now possible to convert peptide release patterns to sequence specificity of proteolytic cleavage

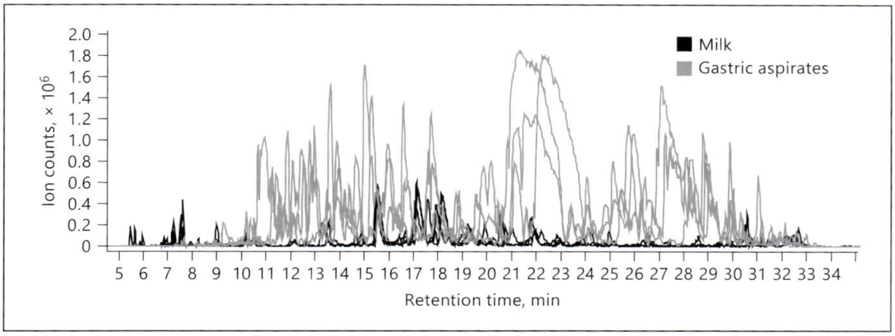

Fig. 1. Ion abundances in intact human milk and gastric aspirates from human infants 1 h after consuming the same human milk. Samples were run on an Agilent (Santa Clara, CA) nano-LC-chip-Q-TOF MS/MS (Chip-Q-TOF) with an Agilent chip C18 column. Total ion abundance extracted chromatograms are shown for representative samples.

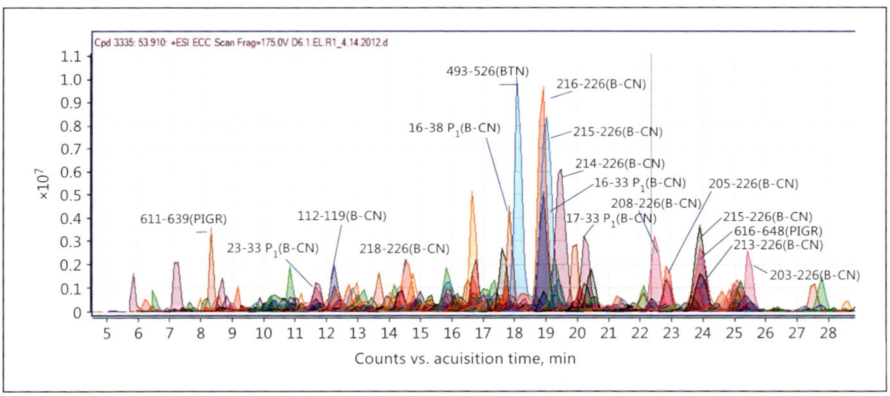

Fig. 2. Annotated ion chromatogram of samples from human stomach aspirates. Peptides were identified by tandem mass spectrometry and mapped to specific proteins according to libraries established through stepwise construction. Samples were run on an Agilent (Santa Clara, CA) nano-LC-chip-Q-TOF MS/MS (Chip-Q-TOF) with an Agilent chip C18 column.

[7, 10]. When this computational strategy is applied to the peptides formed within the stomach of human infants ingesting human milk proteins it is possible to tentatively identify the enzymes that are responsible [10]. Surprisingly, these are not enzymes from the infant but rather enzymes from the milk itself. Transcriptional profiling of mammary epithelial cells documented that the enzymes predicted by computational analyses of peptides were actively expressed as mRNA in the mammary gland [11]. Thus, milk also contains a mixture of

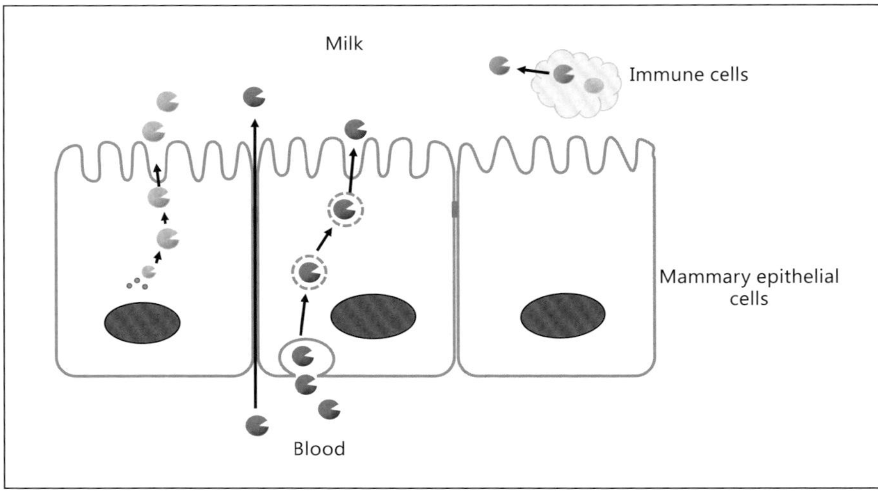

Fig. 3. Schematic of production and transfer of enzymes into milk within the lactating mammary gland. Enzymes can reach milk by direct protein synthesis by the epithelial cell, by translocation from the blood, and via secretion from immune cells within the mammary gland and milk itself.

proteases, zymogens (protease precursors), protease activators, and protease inhibitors, including components of various proteolytic systems such as plasmin, cathepsin, elastase, kallikrein, and amino and carboxypeptidase systems [12]. The basic mechanisms by which enzymes reach milk within the mammary gland are shown in Figure 3.

These studies are confirming that enzymes within the milk contribute to the timing, selectivity, intermediate products, and overall success of protein digestion in the infant stomach and intestine. The advantages to the infant and maternal dyad that drove these aspects of milk through evolutionary pressure remain largely unknown. The value of secreting this complex array of proteolytic system components with milk is a tantalizing example of a dimension of food that is not appreciated, but provides insights into mechanisms by which diet supports the infant's digestive capacity and guides the release of specific and potentially functional peptides.

Implications to Infant Health

A primary role of milk that is well accepted is providing the neonate with high nutritional value proteins. Indeed, research over the past century has documented that milk contains hundreds of proteins, many with identified actions, from antibacterial to immunomodulatory. These components are present in milk due to mammary epithelial cell expression, active or passive transport from blood, or secretion by host immune cells. Now scientific research must incorporate this dimension of selective hydrolysis of milk proteins and the release of specific peptides into our understanding of milk and its value to infant health.

The control of the catalytic activity of the active components of milk such as proteases appears to be complex and multifactorial, including the balance of inhibitors, activators, zymogens, proteases, pH, microlocation, and specific protein structurea of substrates. These milk proteases act on certain proteins, like the caseins but not on others, notably lactoferrin and immunoglobulin. This selectivity means that in vivo some of the milk proteins remain intact to exert their well-known bioactive functions within the infant, and others deliver distinct peptides to sites along the complex biogeography of the infant intestine.

The next phase of research is to understand all of the roles of the milk proteases in vivo. In experiments carried out on infants, they are quantitatively important, and by computation are responsible for the majority of protein degradation within the infant stomach [5, 6]. Studies to date provoke the hypothesis that milk proteases are an evolutionarily driven, beneficial class of milk components that contributes to infant digestive capacity and releases functional peptides that affect infant health. While we have previously assumed that the slow development of the human gastric proteolytic system is a liability to infants, even this assumption may be naïve. As infants have lower digestive capacity than adults [13], the abundance and activity of the proteases of milk exert more control over the digestion of milk itself. The transfer of milk digestion to milk and maternal control implies that the apparent digestive insufficiency of infants has selective advantage as well.

Conclusions

A series of enabling scientific technologies have highlighted the paradoxical properties of milk as a dynamic and biologically active fluid. The breakthroughs that are now emerging on milk emphasize that future research must view the mother-infant dyad as a system of nourishment. Milk needs to be understood for its dynamic nature, its diversity, and its biological activities. Specific peptides are released at specific times into specific sites along the mammary gland and infant intestinal tract. This is possible by virtue of the protein structures in milk, the enzymes that are present, and the ability of the infant to activate those enzymes at specific places and times. Understanding this magnificent system of nourishment is likely to provide insights for nourishing humans of all ages and all health conditions.

Disclosure Statement

Dr. Dallas reports no conflicts of interest. Dr. Dallas's work is supported by the K99/R00 Pathway to Independence Career Award, Eunice Kennedy Shriver Institute of Child Health & Development of the National Institutes of Health (R00HD079561).

Dr. German is a co-founder of Evolve Biosystems a company providing products for breast fed infants. The work is supported by NIH R01AT008759 and R01AT007079.

References

1 Oftedal OT: The mammary gland and its origin during synapsid evolution. J Mammary Gland Biol Neoplasia 2002;7:225–252.

2 Lönnerdal B: Human milk: bioactive proteins/peptides and functional properties; in Bhatia J, Shamir R, Vandenplas Y (eds): Protein in Neonatal and Infant Nutrition: Recent Updates. Nestlé Nutr Inst Workshop Ser. Basel, Karger, 2016, vol 86, pp 97–107.

3 Dallas D, Guerrero A, Khaldi N, et al: Extensive in vivo human milk peptidomics reveals specific proteolysis yielding protective antimicrobial peptides. J Proteome Res 2013;12:2295–2304.

4 Clare DA, Swaisgood HE: Bioactive milk peptides: a prospectus. J Dairy Sci 2000;83:1187–1195.

5 Dallas DC, Guerrero A, Khaldi N, et al: A peptidomic analysis of human milk digestion in the infant stomach reveals protein-specific degradation patterns. J Nutr 2014;144:815–820.

6 Holton TA, Vijayakumar V, Dallas DC, et al: Following the digestion of milk proteins from mother to baby. J Proteome Res 2014;13:5777–5783.

7 Guerrero A, Dallas DC, Contreras S, et al: Mechanistic peptidomics: factors that dictate specificity in the formation of endogenous peptides in human milk. Mol Cell Proteomics 2014;13:3343–3351.

8 Barbano D, Rasmussen R, Lynch J: Influence of milk somatic cell count and milk age on cheese yield. J Dairy Sci 1991;74:369–388.

9 Dallas DC, Guerrero A, Parker EA, et al: Current peptidomics: applications, purification, identification, quantification and functional analysis. Proteomics 2015;15:1026–1038.

10 Khaldi N, Vijayakumar V, Dallas DC, et al: Predicting the important enzymes in human breast milk digestion. J Agric Food Chem 2014;62:7225–7232.

11 Wickramasinghe S, Rincon G, Islas-Trejo A, Medrano JF: Transcriptional profiling of bovine milk using RNA sequencing. BMC Genomics 2012;13:45–58.

12 Dallas DC, Murray NM, Gan J: Proteolytic systems in milk: perspectives on the evolutionary function within the mammary gland and the infant. J Mammary Gland Biol Neoplasia 2015;20:1–15.

13 Dallas DC, Underwood MA, Zivkovic AM, German JB: Digestion of protein in premature and term infants. J Nutr Disord Ther 2012;2:112–121.

Isolauri E, Sherman PM, Walker WA (eds): Intestinal Microbiome: Functional Aspects in Health and Disease. Nestlé Nutr Inst Workshop Ser, vol 88, pp 137–147, (DOI: 10.1159/000455398)

Compositional Analysis and Metabolism of Human Milk Oligosaccharides in Infants

Clemens Kunz[a] • Silvia Rudloff[a, b]

[a]Institute of Nutritional Sciences and [b]Department of Pediatrics, Justus Liebig University Giessen, Giessen, Germany

Abstract

It is a great success that biotechnological means are available today to produce amounts of single human milk oligosaccharides (HMOs) in a purity which allows performing metabolic and functional studies even in humans. As recent data indicate that there is a link between the Lewis blood group and the secretor status of an individual and certain inflammatory diseases, this review will also focus on the metabolic fate of secretor- and Lewis blood group-specific components. We conclude that there is no simple urinary or fecal excretion pattern of HMOs, although the pattern in urine often reflects the mother's secretor/nonsecretor status. However, there are deviations for single HMOs which deserve special attention. In feces, the variation in excretion is much higher than in urine, which may be caused by variations in the infant's intestinal microbiota. A gradual decrease in HMO excretion with time as proposed earlier does not take place as even after 7 months of exclusive breastfeeding often intact HMOs can be detected in feces and urine. In addition, we found that whenever oligosaccharides were detected in feces, LNT, the major core structure of HMOs, was present. Hence, our data do not support speculations that LNT is a preferable source for the microbiota.

Introduction

Already around 1900, concomitant with the discovery of lactobacilli and bifidobacteria and their relevance for health and disease, pediatricians realized that the microbial composition of stool samples from breastfed and bottle-fed infants

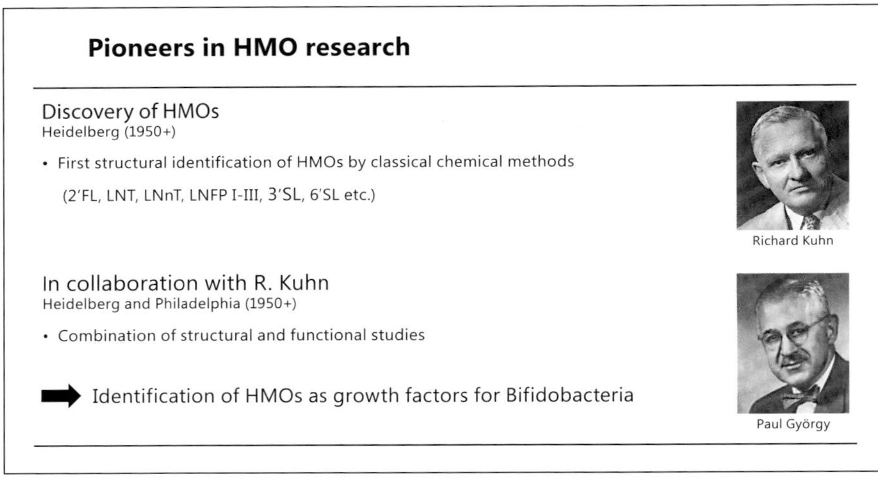

Fig. 1. Discovery of HMOs around 1950 (adapted from Kunz [3]).

differed. Observations indicated that this difference was particularly linked to the milk carbohydrate fraction. This was the starting point of research on human milk carbohydrates. In the middle of the last century, the first human milk oligosaccharides (HMOs) were identified by Richard Kuhn in Heidelberg (Germany) [1]. At the same time, Paul György's studies in Heidelberg and later in Philadelphia (USA) focused on the identification of various HMOs as the "bifidus factor" in human milk (Fig. 1) [2]. Meanwhile about 150–200 single HMOs have been characterized.

In recent years, there has been a tremendous increase in our knowledge regarding specific effects of HMOs [3–10]. Even the first human studies on infant formula supplemented with single HMOs have already been published [11, 12]. In order to determine which compound(s) would be most suitable for supplementation, in which concentrations or combinations, and how long they should be given, studies are needed regarding the metabolic fate of HMOs as well as their local and systemic effects.

A straight forward strategy to investigate the metabolism of HMOs is to determine the presence or absence of natural milk oligosaccharides in feces, blood, urine, or tissue. However, some prerequisites hamper this simple approach as, for example, tissue and blood are not available or rather difficult to obtain from human infants. Also the methodological handling of a large number of samples is still a difficult task and requires standardized methods.

In the following, we briefly address the difficulties of compositional analysis before we present a summary of metabolic aspects from various studies which focus on the excretion of oligosaccharides in feces and urine.

Compositional Analysis of Human Milk Oligosaccharides – Need for Standardized Methods

Standardized methods for routine analysis are not available yet, which is one major reason for the discrepancy between reported qualitative and quantitative data. For the identification of HMOs, various methods such as paper chromatography, HPLC coupled with mass spectrometry (MS), HPAEC-PAD (high-performance anion exchange chromatography), HPLC chip MS, capillary gel electrophoresis/laser-induced fluorescence techniques, or liquid chromatography-HPLC-MS have recently been used. All these methods provide detailed insights into the oligosaccharide pattern of individual milk samples, frequently paired with further information about the relative amount of single isomers. However, most of these techniques require a sophisticated and time-consuming sample preparation, which is a drawback for the analysis of large sample sets.

With regard to quantitative aspects, data from different laboratories also vary significantly [13–17]. Frequently, various MS methods are applied, and concentrations are given as "relative data". However, MS can hardly be recommended for quantitative purposes, and interpretation of those data should be done with caution [18]. In addition, there is the need for using laborious derivatization techniques, such as permethylation or labeling with fluorescence reagents. As a consequence of quantitative considerations, it would be necessary to prove the efficiency of derivatization after each single step. Also, it has to be kept in mind that often a time-consuming sample preparation with various centrifugation and/or extraction steps using different cartridges has to be performed before applying the sample to an MS instrument. The efficiency of those requirements may vary, for example, between individuals or laboratories, issues which should certainly be solved as soon as possible.

Metabolism of Human Milk Oligosaccharides

The high structural diversity of HMOs complicates acquiring a sophisticated knowledge on "what structures are important for infants' health" despite the recent methodological developments to characterize minute amounts of HMOs and their degradation products in biological samples.

Metabolic studies can help to identify if HMOs are absorbed and utilized by the infant's organism. Moreover, fecal oligosaccharide profiling might give an indication of the intestinal health of infants due to the known relationship between microbiota and the abundance of complex glycans in the infant's gut. Urinary excretion can support observations from studies addressing systemic effects of oligosaccharides.

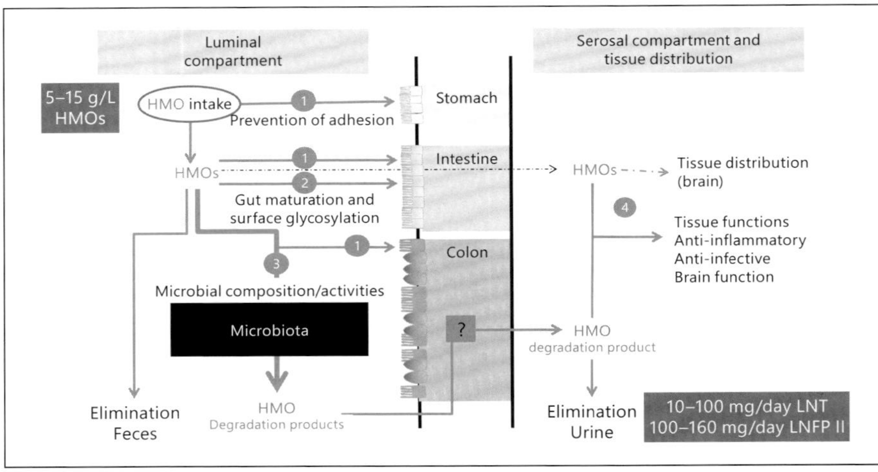

Fig. 2. Intake, metabolism, and potential functions of HMOs. Numbers indicate biological functions, e.g., prevention of pathogen adhesion (1), direct effects on epithelial cells (2), influence on the intestinal microbiota (3), and systemic effects (4) [Modified according to quantitative data from 16, 30].

Only recently, studies trying to prove a direct link between HMO structures and their prebiotic function in vivo in infants have been published. A recent proof-of-concept study indicated an association between the fecal HMO composition and gut microbiota of 2 breastfed infants over time, though both parameters differed substantially between both infants studied [19]. Another study showed a relationship between the fecal microbiome of exclusively breastfed infants and the HMO composition of the milk that was fed [20]. However, since the variation in both (HMOs and microbiota composition) is vast, unequivocal structure-function studies are inevitable for a better understanding of their association with health and disease.

First studies on fecal oligosaccharides and possible metabolites of HMOs in infants have already been reported by Lundblad's group in the 1970s [21]. Recent studies using new technologies either included only one or a low number of infants, or showed data from premature infants whose intestinal function may be very different from healthy term infants [22, 23].

Current data have so far led to the conclusion that the major portion of HMOs reaches the lower gastrointestinal tract where HMOs might be used as nutritive factors by various microorganisms or influence their activities. The remainders are excreted intact or in metabolized form in feces or urine, indicating that there is no uniform metabolic process for all HMOs [5, 24, 25].

Figure 2 shows a summary of the intake, metabolism, and examples for potential functions of HMOs currently being discussed.

Content of Human Milk Oligosaccharides in Term and Preterm Milk

To further improve infant formulas in order to gain more benefit from HMOs, a question often raised is how much of an individual component should be supplemented. In this context, some studies indicated that one has to differentiate between term and preterm milk, as the latter is considered to have either a higher content or a different pattern than term milk [15, 23].

As we recently discussed, we found no difference in the total amount of HMOs between term and preterm milk, neither in colostrum nor in transitory or mature milk, which is exemplified for mature milk in Figure 3a [16].

Often, however, no distinction is made between secretor and nonsecretor milk among the pool of samples analyzed, which will be further discussed in the following.

Intake of Human Milk Oligosaccharides – Differentiation between Lewis Blood Group and Secretor/Nonsecretor Milk Status

It has been established for a long time that the HMO pattern depends on the genetic background of the mother, i.e., on the Lewis blood group and the secretor status (Table 1) [26, 27]. This aspect is particularly important as feeding infants with a different HMO pattern might reduce or even increase the risk for certain diseases.

Grouping the same sample set of term and preterm milk (Figure 3a) according to the secretor status and the Lewis blood group of the mother, it is obvious that there are large differences between milk samples depending on the secretor and Lewis blood group specific pattern (Fig. 3b, c). Differences between individual HMOs in both groups and in Lewis a, Lewis b and Lewis-negative milk samples are further discussed by Kunz et al. [16].

Comparison of Human Milk Oligosaccharides in Milk, Urine, and Feces in Mother-Child Dyads

We performed 2 stable isotope studies collecting milk, feces, urine, and breath samples at each suckling over up to 36 h after having applied an oral bolus of ^{13}C-labeled glucose or galactose given to lactating mothers [28–31]. In the following, we present some of these data together with those from 2 other cohort studies [16, 32].

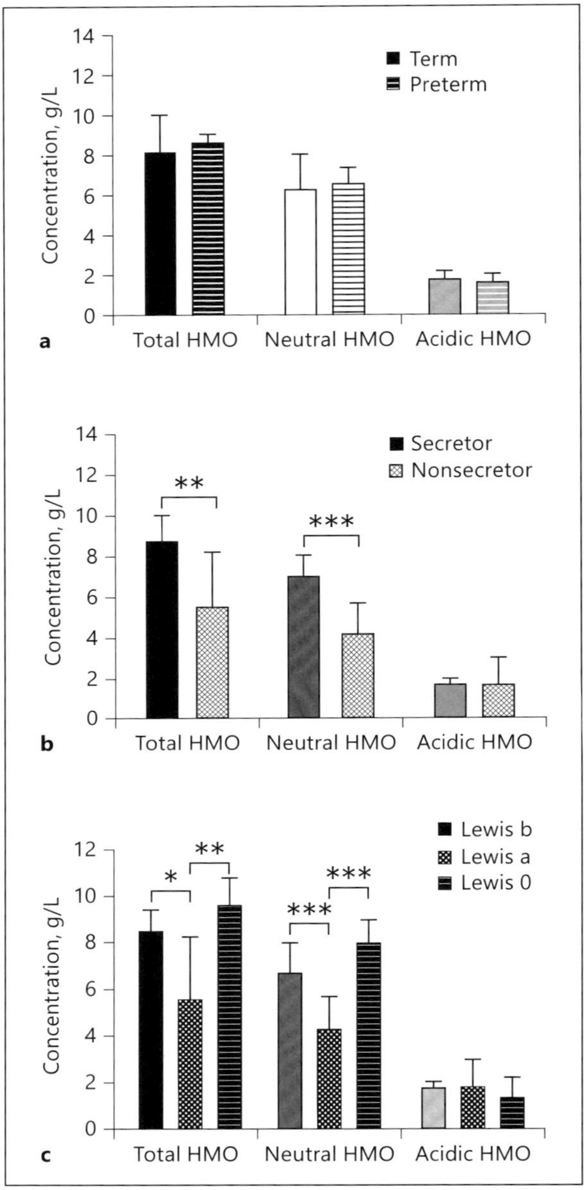

Fig. 3. HMO concentrations in mature human milk from mothers with term or preterm infants (**a**), secretor or nonsecretor status (**b**), and with blood group Lewis a, b, or 0 status (**c**). Concentrations are given as medians and interquartile ranges. * $p < 0.05$; ** $p < 0.01$; *** $p < 0.001$ (adapted from Kunz et al. [16]).

Urinary Excretion Pattern

Our data so far support the general conclusion that the overall pattern of neutral oligosaccharides in the urine from breastfed infants reflects that of their mothers' milk suggesting a strong association with the mothers' Lewis blood

Table 1. Presence of HMO structures according to the Lewis blood group and secretor (sec.) status

HMO structure		Blood group (% of the population)			
name	structure	Lewis b sec. (70)	Lewis a nonsec. (20)	Lewis 0 sec. (5–10)	Lewis 0 nonsec. (0.1–1%)
2'FL	Fuc α_{1-2} Gal β_{1-4} Glc	+	–	+	–
LDFT	Fuc α_{1-2} Gal β_{1-4} (Fuc α_{1-3}) Glc	+	–	+	–
LNFP I	Fuc α_{1-2} Gal β_{1-3} GlcNAc β_{1-3} Gal β_{1-4} Glc	+	–	+	–
LNFP II	Gal β_{1-3} (Fuc α_{1-4}) GlcNac β_{1-3} Gal β_{1-4} Glc	–[1]	+	–[1]	–
LNDFH II	Gal β_{1-3} (Fuc α_{1-4}) GlcNAc β_{1-3} Gal β_{1-4} (Fuc α_{1-3}) Glc	–[1]	+	–[1]	–

2'FL, 2'-fucosyllactose; LDFT, lactodifucotetraose; LNFP, lacto-N-fucopentaose; LNDFH, lacto-N-difucohexaose.
[1] Traces may be present.

group and secretor phenotype. The major difference between the milk from mothers with blood group Lewis a, Lewis b, and Lewis 0 is a rather complex pattern in "Lewis b milk" compared to "Lewis a milk," and "Lewis negative milk" [25, 31, 32, 33]. Comparing HMOs from "Lewis a" or "Lewis b milk" with the urinary oligosaccharide pattern in the corresponding infants, for example, a similar pattern with the same molecular masses was observed [25, 30, 31].

Using MALDI-TOF (matrix assisted laser desorption ionization-time of flight)-MS, differences could be seen in the signal intensities for both, milk and urine, although the masses m/z 730 (LNT, LNnT), 876 (monofucosylated LNT/LNnT), or 1022 (difucosylated LNT/LNnT), as well as others, are present in all samples. As lacto-N-fucopentaose (LNFP) I is characteristic for "Lewis b milk," one would expect that m/z 876, a major mass signal, represents this component; however, MS does not directly allow a clear assignment of various isomeric structures. Analyzing the fraction by HPAEC with pulsed amperometric detection enabling a separation of HMO isomers such as LNFP I and II, we were not able to detect LNFP I in any of the investigated urine samples from infants receiving "Lewis b milk" from their mothers [25, 31].

Fecal Excretion Patterns – Changes with Time

Oligosaccharides known from human milk can be detected in many fecal samples from exclusively breastfed infants [26, 33]. Sometimes the feces of infants displayed a profile distinguishable from milk, where certain HMOs predominated and common, especially larger HMOs, were clearly diminished, and, often, no HMOs were detected, especially after 6–7 months of breastfeeding.

Some infants had reduced abundances of larger structures and a remarkably high proportion of difucosylated LN(n)T (isomers) at *m/z* 1022, which, in contrast, could not be detected in other infants. The predominance of the signal at *m/z* 1022 was also reported by Albrecht et al. [34] in 1 infant. In other cases, however, we observed lower fecal HMO excretions in earlier samples (2 months of age) compared to follow-up samples (7 months of age). This observation is contradictory to the reports of Albrecht et al. [34], who claimed a gradual decrease in HMO abundance with age, hypothesizing an association with gut (microbiota) maturity [22].

Furthermore, one would expect that secretor-specific HMOs would only be present in feces or urine of infants fed milk from "secretor mothers" or "Lewis b mothers." However, we identified secretor-specific oligosaccharides 2′FL, DFLT, and LNDFH I not only in urine and feces from infants fed "secretor milk," but often also in those fed "nonsecretor milk" [25]. This finding is in line with reports by Lundblad's group [21] for feces and the study by De Leoz et al. [35] for urine.

In addition and contradictory to other publications, we detected LNT and LNnT, 2 structures commonly present in human milk, in many infants' urine, and, if HMOs were present, in all fecal samples. In other reports on fecal samples, however, LNT was absent in samples from breastfed infants at different time points [22, 35].

Perspectives

It can be concluded that there is no simple urinary or fecal excretion pattern of HMOs, although the pattern in urine often reflects the mother's secretor/nonsecretor status. However, there are obviously deviations for some single HMOs which deserve special attention. In feces, the variation in excretion is much higher than in urine, which may be caused by variations in the microbial composition within the gastrointestinal tract. A simple gradual decrease in HMO excretion with time as proposed earlier does not take place, as even after 7 months of exclusive breastfeeding intact HMOs can be detected, although in the majority of infants no oligosaccharides are present. In addition, we found that whenever oligosaccharides were detected in feces, LNT, the major core structure of HMOs, was present. Hence, our data do not support previous speculations that LNT is a preferable source for microbiota.

In general, large amounts of HMOs, i.e., several grams per day, reach the gastrointestinal tract of a human milk-fed infant. About 1–5% of HMOs seem to be excreted via infants' urine [19, 28, 29, 31, 36]. Determining the amount of individual HMOs in urine, about 50–160 mg LNT or LNFP II, for example, can be found, a clear indication that HMOs were absorbed [30]. Hence, several hundred milligrams of HMOs per day circulate in the infant's blood. Therefore, it can be expected that not only local effects of HMOs within the gastrointestinal tract but also systemic functions may occur.

Data presented so far raise the question what it means using human milk as the gold standard when it comes to a standard for the composition of HMOs. There are large differences in the total amount and in the pattern of individual HMOs based on the genetic background of the mother. Is the quality of human milk minor when specific HMOs are missing as it is the case in nonsecretors, which comprise about 20% of the population? Do nonsecretor infants deserve special attention assuming that they may have a higher risk for developing certain diseases? Therefore, it may not only be necessary to identify HMOs with the highest benefit for most infants, but also to determine the (health/disease) risk of infants based on their (im)maturity at birth as well as their own genetic background to improve the benefit of HMO supplementation.

Disclosure Statement

There are no conflicts of interest.

References

1 Kuhn R: Les oligosaccharides du lait. Bull Soc Chim Biol 1958;40:297–314.
2 György P: A hitherto unrecognized biochemical difference between human milk and cow's milk. J Pediatr 1953;11:98–108.
3 Kunz C: Historical aspects of human milk oligosaccharides. Adv Nutr 2012;3:430S–439S.
4 Egge H: The diversity of oligosaccharides in human milk; in Renner B, Sawatzki G (eds): New Perspectives in Infant Nutrition. Stuttgart/New York, Thieme, 1993, pp 12–26.
5 Bode L: Human milk oligosaccharides: every baby needs a sugar mama. Glycobiology 2012;22:1147–1162.
6 Asakuma S, Hatakeyama E, Urashima T, et al: Physiology of consumption of human milk oligosaccharides by infant gut-associated bifidobacteria. J Biol Chem 2011;286:34583–34592.
7 Kunz C, Kuntz S, Rudloff S: Bioactivity of human milk oligosaccharides; in Moreno FJ, Sanz ML (eds): Food Oligosaccharides: Production, Analysis and Bioactivity. Oxford, Wiley-Blackwell, 2014, pp 5–20.
8 Sela DA, Mills DA: Nursing our microbiota: molecular linkages between bifidobacteria and milk oligosaccharides. Trends Microbiol 2010;18:298–307.

9 Urashima T, Kitaoka M, Terabayashi T, et al: Milk oligosaccharides; in Gordon NG (ed): Sources, properties and applications. New York, Nova Science Publishers, 2011, pp 1–77.
10 Donovan SM, Wang M, Li M, et al: Host-microbe interactions in the neonatal intestine: role of human milk oligosaccharides. Adv Nutr 2012;3:450S–455S.
11 Marriage BJ, Buck RH, Goehring KC, et al: Infants fed a lower calorie formula with 2′FL show growth and 2′FL uptake like breast-fed infants. J Pediatr Gastroenterol Nutr 2015;61: 649–658.
12 Steenhout P, Sperisen P, Martin F-P, et al: Term infant formula supplemented with human milk oligosaccharides (2′fucosyllactose and lacto-N-neotetraose) shifts stool microbiota and metabolic signature closer to that of breastfed infants (poster). Exp Biol, 2016.
13 Asakuma S, Urashima T, Akahori M, et al: Variation of major neutral oligosaccharides levels in human colostrum. Eur J Clin Nutr 2007;62:488–494.
14 Chaturvedi P, Warren CD, Altaye M, et al: Fucosylated human milk oligosaccharides vary between individuals and over the course of lactation. Glycobiology 2001;11:365–372
15 Gabrielli O, Zampini L, Galeazzi T, et al: Preterm milk oligosaccharides during the first month of lactation. Pediatrics 2011; 128:e1520–e1531.
16 Kunz C, Meyer C, Collado MC, et al: Influence of gestational age, secretor and Lewis blood group status on the oligosaccharide content of human milk. J Pediatr Gastroenterol Nutr, Epub ahead of print.
17 Nakhla T, Fu D, Zopf D, et al: Neutral oligosaccharide content of preterm human milk. Br J Nutr 1999;82:361–367.
18 Duncan MW: Good mass spectrometry and its place in good science. J Mass Spectrom 2012;47:795–809.
19 De Leoz MLA, Kalanetra KM, Bokulich NA, et al: Human milk glycomics and gut microbial genomics in infant feces show a correlation between human milk oligosaccharides and gut microbiota: a proof-of-concept study. J Proteome Res 2015;14:491–502.
20 Wang M, Li M, Wu S, et al: Fecal microbiota composition of breast-fed infants is correlated with human milk oligosaccharides consumed. J Pediatr Gastroenterol Nutr 2015;60: 825–833.
21 Sabharwal H, Nilsson D, Grönberg G, et al: Oligosaccharides from feces of preterm infants fed on breast milk. Arch Biochem Biophys 1988;265:390–406.
22 Albrecht S, Schols HA, Van den Heuvel EGHM, et al: CE-LIF-MS^n profiling of oligosaccharides in human milk and feces of breast-fed babies. Electrophoresis 2010;31: 1264–1273.
23 De Leoz MAL, Gaerlan SC, Strum JS, et al: Lacto-N-tetraose, fucosylation, and secretor status are highly variable in human milk oligosaccharides from women delivering preterm. J Proteome Res 2012;11:4662–4671.
24 Rudloff S, Kunz C: Milk oligosaccharides and metabolism in infants. Adv Nutr 2012;3:398–405.
25 Dotz V, Rudloff S, Meyer C, et al: Metabolic fate of neutral human milk oligosaccharides in exclusively breast-fed infants. Mol Nutr Food Res 2015;59:355–364.
26 Le Pendu J: Histo-blood group antigen and human milk oligosaccharides: genetic polymorphism and risk of infectious diseases. Adv Exp Med Biol 2004;554:135–143.
27 Prieto PA: Profiles of human milk oligosaccharides and production of some human milk oligosaccharides in transgenic animals. Adv Nutr 2012;3:456S–464S.
28 Rudloff S, Pohlentz G, Diekmann L, et al: Urinary excretion of lactose and oligosaccharides in preterm infants fed human milk or infant formula. Acta Paediatr 1996;85:598–603.
29 Rudloff S, Obermeier S, Borsch C, et al: Incorporation of orally applied ^{13}C-galactose into milk lactose and oligosaccharides. Glycobiology 2006;16:477–487.
30 Rudloff S, Pohlentz G, Borsch C, et al: Urinary excretion of in vivo ^{13}C-labelled milk oligosaccharides in breastfed infants. Br J Nutr 2012;107:957–963.
31 Dotz V, Rudloff S, Blank D, et al: ^{13}C-labeled oligosaccharides in breastfed infants' urine: individual-, structure- and time-dependent differences in the excretion. Glycobiology 2014;24:185–194.
32 Dotz V, Adam R, Lochnit G, et al: Neutral oligosaccharides in feces of breastfed and formula-fed infants at different ages. Glycobiology 2016;26:1308–1316.

33 Blank D, Gebhardt S, Maass K, et al: High-throughput mass finger printing and Lewis blood group assignment of human milk oligosaccharides. Anal Bioanal Chem 2011;401: 2495–2510.

34 Albrecht S, Schols HA, van den Heuvel EGHM, et al: Occurrence of oligosaccharides in feces of breast-fed babies in their first six months of life and the corresponding breast milk. Carbohydr Res 2011;346:2540–2550.

35 De Leoz MLA, Wu S, Strum JS, et al: A quantitative and comprehensive method to analyze human milk oligosaccharide structures in the urine and feces of infants. Anal Bioanal Chem 2013;405:4089–4105.

36 Goehring KC, Kennedy AD, Prieto PA: Direct evidence for the presence of human milk oligosaccharides in the circulation of breast-fed infants. PLoS One 2014;9:e101692.

37 Rose CS, Kuhn R, Zilliken F, Gyorgy P: Bifidus factor. V. The activity of α- and β-methyl-N-acetyl-D-glucosaminides. Arch Biochem Biophys 1954;49:123–129.

Isolauri E, Sherman PM, Walker WA (eds): Intestinal Microbiome: Functional Aspects in Health and Disease. Nestlé Nutr Inst Workshop Ser, vol 88, pp 149–159, (DOI: 10.1159/000455399)
Nestec Ltd., Vevey/S. Karger AG., Basel, © 2017

Differential Establishment of Bifidobacteria in the Breastfed Infant Gut

Zachery T. Lewis[a, b] · David A. Mills[a–c]

[a]Foods for Health Institute, and [b]Departments of Food Science and Technology and [c]Viticulture and Enology, University of California Davis, Davis, CA, USA

Abstract

The composition of an infant's gut microbiome can impact their immediate and long-term health. Bifdobacteria play a major role in structuring the gut microbiome of breastfed infants due to their ability to consume oligosaccharides found in human milk. However, recent studies have revealed that bifidobacteria are often absent in the gut microbiome of breastfed infants in some locations. This lack of colonization may be due either to differences in the environmental conditions in the gastrointestinal tract of uncolonized infants which prohibit the growth of bifidobacteria or a dearth of sources from which infants may acquire these specialized bacterial species. Potential mechanisms by which these broad factors may lead to lower colonization of infants by bifidobacteria are discussed herein. Environmental conditions which may select against bifidobacteria include low rates/duration of breastfeeding, milk glycan composition, and antimicrobial use. Routes of colonization by bifidobacteria which may be disrupted include maternal transfer via vaginal birth, fecal-oral routes, or via breast milk itself. A careful contemplation of the conditions experienced by bifidobacteria over human evolutionary history may lead to further hypotheses as to the causative factors of the differential colonization by this foundation genus in some contemporary locations.

Introduction

Breastfeeding benefits human infants in numerous ways. One realm in which breast milk exerts an influence is in the development of the infant intestinal microbiome. Infants transition from near sterility in the womb to a sudden embrace by the microbial diversity of their new ex utero environment and yet possess a gut microbiota temporarily distinct from that of adults who encounter many of the same sources of inoculum. The guts of breastfed infants are typically dominated by bifidobacteria, unlike those of adults [1, 2]. Bifidobacteria are gram-positive anaerophilic bacteria commonly used as probiotics and are beneficial to infants in a number of ways. Infants with bifidobacteria-dominated gastrointestinal tracts are more resistant to colonization by pathogens, respond better to some vaccines, and possess better-functioning gut barriers [3–6]. Bifidobacteria also appear to simultaneously enhance immune surveillance and reduce inflammation [6–9]. Infant-type bifidobacteria present during weaning may guide the immune system towards tolerance during the introduction of new foods and their associated antigens, potentially influencing the development of allergic diseases [10–13]. For these public health reasons, among other motivations, bifidobacterial levels have been studied in infants across the globe.

Interestingly, it seems that not all infants have large amounts of bifidobacteria in their stool [14]. Comparisons of worldwide datasets (Norway [15], Sweden [16], Canada [17], Italy [18], Switzerland [19], Bangladesh [4], the USA [20], Malawi, and Finland [21]) show that the gut microbiomes of healthy breastfed infants in some populations had lower amounts of bifidobacteria than others. While further study is needed on the importance of bifidobacterial colonization in infants from such diverse contexts, given the apparent benefits of their presence, identifying the cause(s) of this phenomenon and developing potential solutions is of interest. The Dutch microbiologist Lourens Baas Becking once famously hypothesized that when it came to microbial biogeography "Everything is everywhere, but the environment selects" [22]. Proposed mechanisms for the differential bifidobacterial abundance phenomenon may be broken down into two broad categories mirroring Bass Becking's statement: either the gut environments of some infants are differentially selective (against bifidobacteria), or there are higher barriers to bifidobacteria getting into infants in some places than others (bifidobacteria are, in fact, not "everywhere"). Using this conceptual framework, we will discuss various hypotheses for how bifidobacteria are acquired by infants, and how the gut microbiota is shaped in ways that may impact the immediate and future health of an infant.

Environmental Selection in the Gut

Many factors that influence the gut microbiome of infants fall under the general umbrella of selection-based determination, including the antimicrobial ingredients of breast milk (lysozyme, lactoferrin, and antibodies), the infant immune system, and infant exposure to antimicrobials [23–25]. Antibiotic use in particular has been recently shown to impact the infant microbiome, with some studies indicating that antibiotic exposure lowers bifidobacterial levels [26–29]. However, of the potential environmental conditions exerting selective pressure on the gut microbiota, diet is perhaps the most apparent, both in adults and infants [17, 30, 31]. Breast milk has been the principal source of nutrition for infants over human evolutionary history, and formula feeding leads to disruptions in the typical pattern of microbiota development in infants [30, 32]. The mechanism by which breast milk influences the microbiota is of translational interest, as current diet-based means to alter microbial ecosystems in a targeted manner are poorly developed. Breast milk contains macronutrient concentrations of oligosaccharides and glycoconjugates, collectively known as human milk glycans (HMGs) [33]. These carbohydrates pass undigested through the infant small intestine, and, once in the colon, they act as prebiotics supporting the establishment of bifidobacteria [34].

Select bifidobacterial species are uniquely equipped to fully consume the complex HMGs found in breast milk [35]. For example, *Bifidobacterium longum* subsp. *infantis* colonized premature infants better than *Bifidobacterium animalis* subsp. *lactis* when given concurrently with human milk, likely due to the capacity of *B. longum* subsp. *infantis* to consume a wider variety of HMGs [36, 37]. The structural complexity of HMGs serves as a barrier to other microbes which cannot successfully compete with bifidobacteria specialized for growth on these substrates. It should also be noted that not all breast milk contains the same mixture of HMGs. For example, maternal secretor status can influence the amount and type of fucosylated oligosaccharides present, which impacts the microbial community structure [20]. In this way, a breast milk diet is selective for a narrow set of bacterial species. The selective pressures of breast milk are strong enough that it is the cessation of breastfeeding, rather than the introduction of complementary foods, that allows for a community-wide shift in microbial composition [38]. Given this knowledge, it is plausible that cultural differences in the duration or rates of breastfeeding between locations may lead to differential colonization by bifidobacteria due to the availability of these selective growth substrates.

The context of other species present in any given infant is also an important selective factor in shaping the final community and thus infant health. Microbes do not exist in isolation but in consortia with large numbers of different taxa, which cooperate and compete in a dizzying array of interactions. *Bacteroides* and bifidobacteria, for example, have strain level metabolic interactions which depend on carbon source availability [39, 40]. They can both consume at least some HMGs, though select bifidobacteria have been shown to outcompete

Bacteroides for these growth substrates [41]. In the absence of HMG-consuming bifidobacteria, however, *Bacteroides* species may dominate the infant gut microbiome and expose the infant to increased amounts of lipopolysaccharide types which are linked to downstream autoimmune disease [42]. In addition, *Bacteroides* degradation products of sialylated milk oligosaccharides have been shown to promote the growth of potentially pathogenic Enterobacteriaceae in in vitro studies, suggesting the presence of a "cross-feeding" effect [43–45]. This outgrowth of Enterobacteriaceae may also induce gut inflammation [45]. Several studies have previously observed a trade-off between the abundance of bifidobacteria and Proteobacteria in infants, which may partially be the result of the import-and-degrade strategy of HMG consumption of some bifidobacteria, which, unlike *Bacteroides*, do not leave behind degradation products for future proteobacterial consumption [4, 20, 37, 46] (Fig. 1). Some bifidobacteria do externally degrade glycans, as *Bifidobacterium bifidum* deploys external glycosyl hydrolases which have been shown to promote cross-feeding [47].

The metabolic end products of bifidobacterial metabolism (i.e. lactate and acetate) can also feed and influence the rest of the microbial community [48]. Acetate is also known to be protective against some pathogens [3]. Acetate and lactate also have the secondary effect of lowering the pH of the fecal environment, which is in and of itself a major selective factor, including via specific inhibition of *Bacteroides* species [49–51]. Taken together, this evidence suggests that colonization of breastfed infants by HMG-consuming bifidobacteria averts an alternative pattern of microbiota establishment which may include overexposure to *Bacteroides* endotoxin, cross-feeding of potentially pathogenic Enterobacteriaceae, and the induction of proinflammatory cytokines – all of which impact infant health.

Acquisition of Species: Bacterial Migration and Transmission

In comparison to environmental selection, the transmission of microbial species to the infant gastrointestinal tract is more difficult to measure. Many studies show overlap between operational taxonomic units in putative source environments and the infant gut microbiome, but this does not show directionality of transfer, nor does it rule out a third common source for the other two environments. However, there is existing evidence to support several possible routes of transfer to at least some infants.

The initial source of microbes in infants is often thought to be from the mother. The placenta is near sterile and likely contributes little to the gut microbiome in the first days of life [52]. Transfer from the mother's vaginal canal during birth

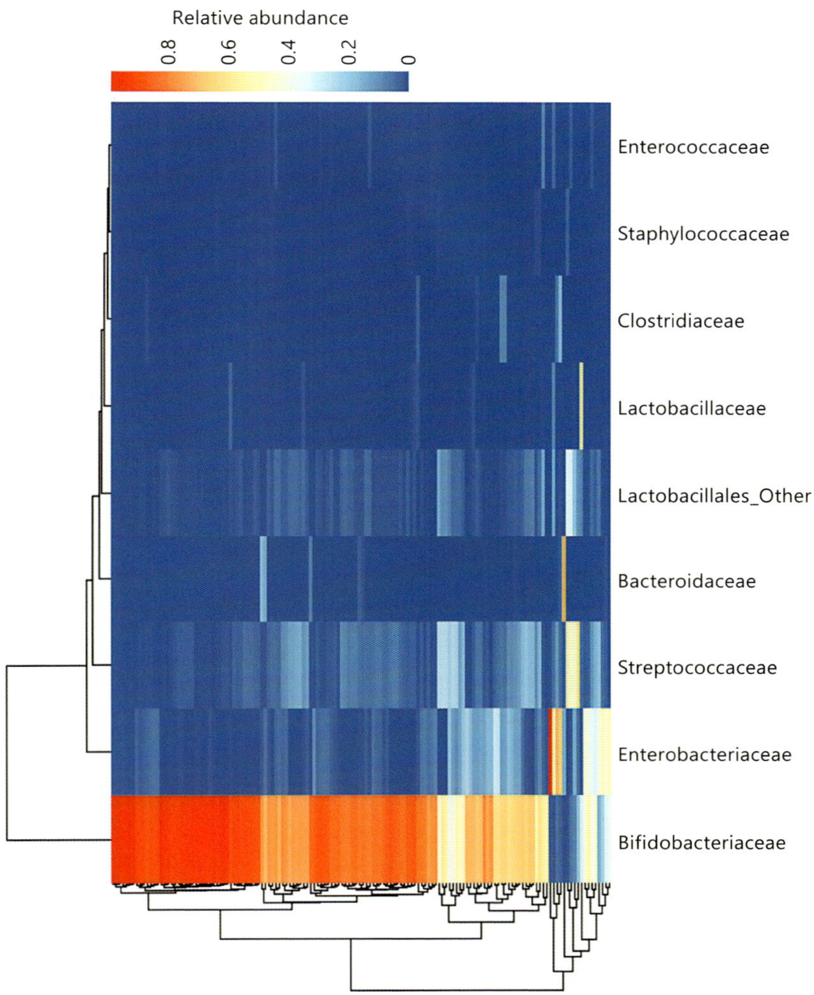

Fig. 1. Trade-off between the abundances of bifidobacteria and *Bacteroides* in the gut of breastfed infants: the gut microbial community of infants in Bangladesh (adapted from Huda et al. [4]). Samples in rows are clustered by microbiome euclidean distance using a complete agglomeration method. Samples are colored in each column according to the relative abundance of the microbe on the *x*-axis label in that sample (1 = 100% abundance). Bifidobacteria dominate the gut microbiome of most infants and appear to be mutually exclusive with Enterobacteriaceae and Bacteroidaceae.

is the first major source of inoculum [53]. Cesarean section birth limits exposure to possible inoculation both via maternal stool during birth and via vaginal contact, and, as a result, cesarean section-born infants often possess distinct gut microbial assemblages which are occasionally lower in bifidobacteria [17, 32, 54]. Bifidobacteria have been detected in the vagina, although specialized HMG degraders such as *B. longum* subsp. *infantis* appear to be rare in that environment, and, where found, their presence may be due to fecal contamination [55–59]. The mother's intestinal microbiota is a likely source of some bifidobacteria for the infant, both during and after the birthing process, and several studies have proven strain congruence among isolates from mother's and infant's feces [55, 60]. The skin of mothers and other caretakers may also be a vector for the early transfer of intestinal microbes [61]. Other potential sources of microbes include siblings, pets, and the built environment [62–64].

Breast milk contains microbes, including bifidobacteria, but their origin and potential impact on colonization remains unclear [65–68]. Reverse flow of milk during nursing indicates likely contaminating transfer of external microbes into the mammary gland, complicating inference of transfer directionality [69]. A so-called "enteromammary" pathway has also been postulated whereby the mother's immune system gathers microbes from the mother's gastrointestinal tract and, without killing them, transfers them to be expressed from the mammary gland to the infant during suckling at the breast [70, 71]. This hypothesis remains speculative and has the disadvantage that the absolute number of microbes transferred in such a system would likely be relatively low in comparison to inoculation from other sources (i.e., feces). Whether an elaborate system for transferring what were likely common infant intestinal microbes would be advantageous in the "environment of evolutionary adaptedness" [72] (the ancestral conditions under which the proposed enteromammary pathway putatively arose) or whether a simple fecal-oral route would suffice is an open question.

The environment of evolutionary adaptedness was likely more microbially intensive than is typical in developed nations today, given the lack of hygiene, absence of man-made antimicrobials, and more regular exposure to the diverse array of "outdoor" microbes that go hand-in-hand with a hunter-gatherer or, later, pastoral lifestyle [73]. However, anaerophilic HMG-degrading specialist bifidobacteria were and are not likely to be ubiquitous in all putative source environments for intestinal microbes. Indeed, bifidobacteria have been rare in the gastrointestinal tract of human adults in the traditionally living people studied so far [74]. Indeed, *Bifidobacterium* abundance in adults appears to correlate with the consumption of dairy in the population, as the genus is absent from the Hadza hunter-gatherers (no access to dairy) while being prevalent only in the urban populations of the remote Nicobarese tribe (the subpopulation which has access to dairy) [75, 76]. However, it is often difficult to disentangle the effect of dairy with that of simply living in higher-density populations with more opportunity for horizontal acquisition of microbes from other individuals. The ultimate source of infant-type bifidobacteria, for the moment, remains unidentified.

Conclusion

The past century has seen drastic shifts in both the selective pressures experienced by the human gut microbiota and the opportunities for microbe transmission. The possibility for undesirable side effects of these changes has recently become increasingly clear. Lack of exposure to commensal species, such as bifidobacteria, was unlikely to be an issue often faced by our ancestors. Human physiology may have co-evolved with "expected" exposure to bifidobacteria during the life stages concurrent with breastfeeding, and their presence may provide important developmental cues and protection from disease. Because bifidobacteria are an important foundation species that unlock a key carbon source and facilitate an entire metabolic network leading to adaptive development of the infant gut microbiota, their disappearance may lead to sequelae of public health importance [71, 77, 78]. The "hygiene hypothesis" encompasses this idea and attempts to connect diseases such as diabetes, inflammatory bowel disease, autism, allergies, atopy, metabolic syndrome, and chronic inflammatory bowel diseases with microbial dysbiosis [reviewed in 11, 71, 79].

To design interventions that remedy putative *Bifidobacterium*-related microbial dysbiosis early in life and avoid its potential undesirable outcomes, one must first understand the reasons behind the undercolonization of infants by bifidobacteria in some locations. If the causative mechanism falls under the "environmental selection" umbrella, the solution would need to shift conditions in the gut, such as eliminating the presence of antimicrobials or promoting bifidobacterial growth through targeted HMG-like prebiotics. If the cause is instead that many infants are simply never exposed to the appropriate bifidobacteria, application of an HMG-consuming *Bifidobacterium*-containing probiotic may be a simple solution. However, no amount of prebiotic can enrich a taxa that is not present, and no amount of administered live bifidobacterial cells can establish colonization of a species in an environment that is nonpermissive for its growth. Transnational comparisons of breastfed infant gut microbial communities, combined with the appropriate metadata, may be useful to disentangle the relevant contributing factors and clarify what drives local bifidobacterial colonization patterns. Such studies may best be conducted in the form of ongoing "microbial community observatories" as suggested by Charbonneau et al. [80]. Ultimately, the combination of multiple types of expertise, such as anthropology, epidemiology, microbiology, chemistry, medicine, and public health, will be necessary to address this developing phenomenon.

Acknowledgments

We kindly thank Steven Frese for his assistance with Figure 1. This work was supported, in part, by funding from National Institutes of Health awards R01AT007079 and R01AT008759 and the Peter J. Shields Endowed Chair in Dairy Food Science (D.A.M.). Z.T.L. is supported by an Alfred P. Sloan Foundation's Microbiology of the Built Environment postdoctoral fellowship.

Disclosure Statement

D.A.M. is a co-founder of Evolve Biosystems, a company focused on diet-based manipulation of the gut microbiota. Evolve BioSystems played no role in the design, execution, interpretation, or publication of this study.

References

1 Yatsunenko T, Rey FE, Manary MJ, et al: Human gut microbiome viewed across age and geography. Nature 2012;486:222–227.

2 Khonsari S, Suganthy M, Burczynska B, et al: A comparative study of bifidobacteria in human babies and adults. Biosci Microbiota 2016;35:97–103.

3 Fukuda S, Toh H, Hase K, et al: Bifidobacteria can protect from enteropathogenic infection through production of acetate. Nature 2011;469:543–547.

4 Huda MN, Lewis ZT, Kalanetra KM, et al: Stool microbiota and vaccine responses of infants. Pediatrics 2014;134:e362–e372.

5 Romond M-B, Colavizza M, Mullié C, et al: Does the intestinal bifidobacterial colonisation affect bacterial translocation? Anaerobe 2008;14:43–48.

6 Chichlowski M, De Lartigue G, German JB, et al: Bifidobacteria isolated from infants and cultured on human milk oligosaccharides affect intestinal epithelial function. J Pediatr Gastroenterol Nutr 2012;55:321–327.

7 Sheil B, MacSharry J, O'Callaghan L, et al: Role of interleukin (IL-10) in probiotic-mediated immune modulation: an assessment in wild-type and IL-10 knock-out mice. Clin Exp Immunol 2006;144:273–280.

8 Tanabe S, Kinuta Y, Saito Y: *Bifidobacterium infantis* suppresses proinflammatory interleukin-17 production in murine splenocytes and dextran sodium sulfate-induced intestinal inflammation. Int J Mol Med 2008;22: 181–185.

9 Preising J, Philippe D, Gleinser M, et al: Selection of bifidobacteria based on adhesion and anti-inflammatory capacity in vitro for amelioration of murine colitis. Appl Environ Microbiol 2010;76:3048–3051.

10 Young SL, Simon MA, Baird MA, et al: Bifidobacterial species differentially affect expression of cell surface markers and cytokines of dendritic cells harvested from cord blood. Clin Diagn Lab Immunol 2004;11:686–690.

11 Brown EM, Arrieta M-C, Finlay BB: A fresh look at the hygiene hypothesis: how intestinal microbial exposure drives immune effector responses in atopic disease. Semin Immunol 2013;25:378–387.
12 Kirjavainen P V, Arvola T, Salminen SJ, Isolauri E: Aberrant composition of gut microbiota of allergic infants: a target of bifidobacterial therapy at weaning? Gut 2002;51: 51–55.
13 Enomoto T, Sowa M, Nishimori K, et al: Effects of bifidobacterial supplementation to pregnant women and infants in the prevention of allergy development in infants and on fecal microbiota. Allergol Int 2014;63:575–585.
14 Tannock GW, Lee PS, Wong KH, et al: Why don't all infants have bifidobacteria in their stool? Front Microbiol 2016;7:834.
15 Avershina E, Ola S, Oien T, et al: Major fecal microbiota shifts in composition and diversity with age in a geographically restricted cohort of mothers and their children. FEMS Microbiol Ecol 2014;87:280–290.
16 Abrahamsson TR, Jakobsson HE, Andersson AF, et al: Low gut microbiota diversity in early infancy precedes asthma at school age. Clin Exp Allergy 2014;44:842–850.
17 Azad MB, Konya T, Maughan H, et al: Gut microbiota of healthy Canadian infants: profiles by mode of delivery and infant diet at 4 months. CMAJ 2013;185:385–394.
18 Roos S, Dicksved J, Tarasco V, et al: 454 pyrosequencing analysis on faecal samples from a randomized DBPC trial of colicky infants treated with *Lactobacillus reuteri* DSM 17938. PLoS One 2013;8:e56710.
19 Jost T, Lacroix C, Braegger CP, Chassard C: New insights in gut microbiota establishment in healthy breast fed neonates. PLoS One 2012;7:e44595.
20 Lewis ZT, Totten SM, Smilowitz JT, et al: Maternal fucosyltransferase 2 status affects the gut bifidobacterial communities of breastfed infants. Microbiome 2015;3:1–21.
21 Grześkowiak Ł, Collado MC, Mangani C, et al: Distinct gut microbiota in southeastern African and northern European infants. J Pediatr Gastroenterol Nutr 2012;54:812–816.
22 de Wit R, Bouvier T: "Everything is everywhere, but, the environment selects," what did Baas Becking and Beijerinck really say? Environ Microbiol 2006;8:755–758.
23 Microbiomes H, Halden RU: Lessons learned from probing for impacts of triclosan and triclocarban on human microbiomes. mSphere 2014;1:1–4.
24 Zivkovic AM, Lewis ZT, German JB, Mills DA: Establishment of a milk-oriented microbiota (MOM) in early life: how babies meet their MOMs. Funct Food Rev 2013;5:3–12.
25 van Best N, Hornef MW, Savelkoul PHM, Penders J: On the origin of species: factors shaping the establishment of infant's gut microbiota. Birth Defects Res Part C Embryo Today 2015;105:240–251.
26 Korpela K, Salonen A, Virta LJ, et al: Association of early-life antibiotic use and protective effects of breastfeeding: role of the intestinal microbiota. JAMA Pediatr 2016;170:750–757.
27 Yassour M, Vatanen T, Siljander H, et al: Natural history of the infant gut microbiome and impact of antibiotic treatment on bacterial strain diversity and stability. Sci Transl Med 2016;8:343ra81.
28 Bokulich NA, Chung J, Battaglia T, et al: Antibiotics, birth mode, and diet shape microbiome maturation during early life. Sci Transl Med 2016;8:343ra82 .
29 Azad M, Konya T, Persaud R, et al: Impact of maternal intrapartum antibiotics, method of birth and breastfeeding on gut microbiota during the first year of life: a prospective cohort study. BJOG 2015;123:983–993.
30 Liu Z, Roy NC, Guo Y, et al: Human breast milk and infant formulas differentially modify the intestinal microbiota in human infants and host physiology in rats. J Nutr 2016;146: 191–199.
31 Muegge BD, Kuczynski J, Knights D, et al: Diet drives convergence in gut microbiome functions across mammalian phylogeny and within humans. Science 2011;332:970–974.
32 Madan JC, Hoen AG, Lundgren SN, et al: Association of cesarean delivery and formula supplementation with the intestinal microbiome of 6-week-old infants. JAMA Pediatr 2016;170:212–219.
33 German JB, Freeman SL, Lebrilla CB, Mills DA: Human milk oligosaccharides: evolution, structures and bioselectivity as substrates for intestinal bacteria. Nestle Nutr Work Ser Pediatr Progr 2008;62:205–222.
34 Kunz C, Rudloff S, Baier W, et al: Oligosaccharides in human milk: structural, functional, and metabolic aspects. Annu Rev Nutr 2000;20:699–722.

35 Garrido D, Dallas DC, Mills DA: Consumption of human milk glycoconjugates by infant-associated bifidobacteria: mechanisms and implications. Microbiology 2013;159: 649–664.
36 LoCascio RG, Desai P, Sela DA, et al: Broad conservation of milk utilization genes in *Bifidobacterium longum* subsp. *infantis* as revealed by comparative genomic hybridization. Appl Environ Microbiol 2010;76: 7373–7381.
37 Underwood MA, Kalanetra KM, Bokulich NA, et al: A comparison of two probiotic strains of bifidobacteria in premature infants. J Pediatr 2013;163:1585–1591.
38 Bäckhed F, Roswall J, Peng Y, et al: Dynamics and stabilization of the human gut microbiome during the first year of life. Cell Host Microbe 2015;17:690–703.
39 Rios-Covian D, Arboleya S, Hernandez-Barranco AM, et al: Interactions between *Bifidobacterium* and *Bacteroides* species in cofermentations are affected by carbon sources, including exopolysaccharides produced by bifidobacteria. Appl Environ Microbiol 2013; 79:7518–7524.
40 Falony G, Calmeyn T, Leroy F, De Vuyst L: Coculture fermentations of *Bifidobacterium* species and *Bacteroides thetaiotaomicron* reveal a mechanistic insight into the prebiotic effect of inulin-type fructans. Appl Environ Microbiol 2009;75:2312–2319.
41 Marcobal A, Barboza M, Sonnenburg ED, et al: *Bacteroides* in the infant gut consume milk oligosaccharides via mucus-utilization pathways. Cell Host Microbe 2011;10:507–514.
42 Vatanen T, Kostic AD, d'Hennezel E, et al: Variation in microbiome LPS immunogenicity contributes to autoimmunity in humans. Cell 2016;165:1551.
43 Charbonneau MR, O'Donnell D, Blanton LV, et al: Sialylated milk oligosaccharides promote microbiota-dependent growth in models of infant undernutrition. Cell 2016;164: 1–13.
44 Frese SA, Parker K, Calvert CC, Mills DA: Diet shapes the gut microbiome of pigs during nursing and weaning. Microbiome 2015; 3:28.
45 Huang Y-L, Chassard C, Hausmann M, et al: Sialic acid catabolism drives intestinal inflammation and microbial dysbiosis in mice. Nat Commun 2015;6:8141.
46 Wang M, Li M, Wu S, et al: Fecal microbiota composition of breast-fed infants is correlated with human milk oligosaccharides consumed. J Pediatr Gastroenterol Nutr 2015;60: 825–833.
47 Egan M, Motherway MO, Kilcoyne M, et al: Cross-feeding by *Bifidobacterium breve* UCC2003 during co-cultivation with *Bifidobacterium bifidum* PRL2010 in a mucin-based medium. BMC Microbiol 2014;14:282.
48 De Vuyst L, Leroy F: Cross-feeding between bifidobacteria and butyrate-producing colon bacteria explains bifdobacterial competitiveness, butyrate production, and gas production. Int J Food Microbiol 2011;149:73–80.
49 Ogawa K, Ben RA, Pons S, et al: Volatile fatty acids, lactic acid, and pH in the stools of breast-fed and bottle-fed infants. J Pediatr Gastroenterol Nutr 1992;15:248–252.
50 Lauber CL, Hamady M, Knight R, Fierer N: Pyrosequencing-based assessment of soil pH as a predictor of soil bacterial community structure at the continental scale. Appl Environ Microbiol 2009;75:5111–5120.
51 Walker AW, Duncan SH, Leitch ECM, et al: pH and peptide supply can radically alter bacterial populations and short-chain fatty acid ratios within microbial communities from the human colon. Appl Environ Microbiol 2005;71:3692–3700.
52 Lauder AP, Roche AM, Sherrill-Mix S, et al: Comparison of placenta samples with contamination controls does not provide evidence for a distinct placenta microbiota. Microbiome 2016;4:29.
53 Dominguez-Bello MG, Costello EK, Contreras M, et al: Delivery mode shapes the acquisition and structure of the initial microbiota across multiple body habitats in newborns. Proc Natl Acad Sci U S A 2010;107:11971–11975.
54 Martin R, Makino H, Cetinyurek Yavuz A, et al: Early-life events, including mode of delivery and type of feeding, siblings and gender, shape the developing gut microbiota. PLoS One 2016;11:e0158498.
55 Mikami K, Takahashi H, Kimura M, et al: Influence of maternal bifidobacteria on the establishment of bifidobacteria colonizing the gut in infants. Pediatr Res 2009;65:669–674.

56 Makino H, Kushiro A, Ishikawa E, et al: Transmission of intestinal *Bifidobacterium longum* subsp. *longum* strains from mother to infant, determined by multilocus sequencing typing and amplified fragment length polymorphism. Appl Environ Microbiol 2011;77: 6788–6793.
57 Makino H, Kushiro A, Ishikawa E, et al: Mother-to-infant transmission of intestinal bifidobacterial strains has an impact on the early development of vaginally delivered infant's microbiota. PLoS One 2013;8:e78331.
58 Burton JP, Dixon JL, Reid G: Detection of *Bifidobacterium* species and *Gardnerella vaginalis* in the vagina using PCR and denaturing gradient gel electrophoresis. 2003;81:61–63.
59 Chaban B, Links MG, Jayaprakash TP, et al: Characterization of the vaginal microbiota of healthy Canadian women through the menstrual cycle. Microbiome 2014;2:23.
60 Fanaro S, Chierici R, Guerrini P, Vigi V: Intestinal microflora in early infancy: composition and development. Acta Paediatr Suppl 2003;91:48–55.
61 Adlerberth I, Wold AE: Establishment of the gut microbiota in Western infants. Acta Paediatr 2009;98:229–238.
62 Lax S, Smith D, Shogan BD, et al: Longitudinal analysis of microbial interaction between humans and the indoor environment. Science 2014;345:1048–1052.
63 Song SJ, Lauber C, Costello EK, et al: Cohabiting family members share microbiota with one another and with their dogs. eLIFE 2013; 2:e00458.
64 Konya T, Koster B, Maughan H, et al: Associations between bacterial communities of house dust and infant gut. Environ Res 2014; 131:25–30.
65 Perez PF, Doré J, Leclerc M, et al: Bacterial imprinting of the neonatal immune system: lessons from maternal cells? Pediatrics 2007; 119:e724–e732.
66 Fernández L, Langa S, Martín V, et al: The human milk microbiota: origin and potential roles in health and disease. Pharmacol Res 2013;69:1–10.
67 Urbaniak C, Burton JP, Reid G: Breast, milk and microbes: a complex relationship that does not end with lactation. Womens Health (Lond) 2012;8:385–398.
68 Martín R, Jiménez E, Heilig H, et al: Isolation of bifidobacteria from breast milk and assessment of the bifidobacterial population by PCR-denaturing gradient gel electrophoresis and quantitative real-time PCR. Appl Environ Microbiol 2009;75:965–969.
69 Ramsay DT, Kent JC, Owens RA, Hartmann PE: Ultrasound imaging of milk ejection in the breast of lactating women. Pediatrics 2004;113:361–367.
70 Jeurink PV, van Bergenhenegouwen J, Jiménez E, et al: Human milk: a source of more life than we imagine. Benef Microbes 2013;4: 17–30.
71 Scholtens PAMJ, Oozeer R, Martin R, et al: The early settlers: intestinal microbiology in early life. Annu Rev Food Sci Technol 2012;3: 425–447.
72 Bowlby J: Attachment and Loss. New York, Basic Books, 1969.
73 Schnorr SL: The diverse microbiome of the hunter-gatherer. Nature 2015;518:S14.
74 Obregon-Tito AJ, Tito RY, Metcalf J, et al: Subsistence strategies in traditional societies distinguish gut microbiomes. Nat Commun 2015;6:6505.
75 Schnorr SL, Candela M, Rampelli S, et al: Gut microbiome of the Hadza hunter-gatherers. Nat Commun 2014;5:3654.
76 Anwesh M, Kumar KV, Nagarajan M, et al: Elucidating the richness of bacterial groups in the gut of Nicobarese tribal community – perspective on their lifestyle transition. Anaerobe 2016;39:68–76.
77 Biasucci G, Benenati B, Morelli L, et al: Cesarean delivery may affect the early biodiversity of intestinal bacteria. J Nutr 2008;138: 1796S–1800S.
78 Sassone-Corsi M, Raffatellu M: No vacancy: how beneficial microbes cooperate with immunity to provide colonization resistance to pathogens. J Immunol 2015;194:4081–4087.
79 Bäckhed F, Fraser CM, Ringel Y, et al: Defining a healthy human gut microbiome: current concepts, future directions, and clinical applications. Cell Host Microbe 2012;12:611–622.
80 Charbonneau MR, Blanton LV, DiGiulio DB, et al: A microbial perspective of human developmental biology. Nature 2016;535:48–55.

Isolauri E, Sherman PM, Walker WA (eds): Intestinal Microbiome: Functional Aspects in Health and Disease. Nestlé Nutr Inst Workshop Ser, vol 88, pp 161–170, (DOI: 10.1159/000455400)
Nestec Ltd., Vevey/S. Karger AG., Basel, © 2017

Regulatory Aspects of Human Milk Oligosaccharides

Seppo Salminen

Functional Foods Forum, Faculty of Medicine, University of Turku, Turku, Finland

Abstract

Human milk oligosaccharides are key components of human milk and appear in various compositions and concentrations in all human milks. In regulatory sense human milk oligosaccharides are classified as novel foods or novel food ingredients requiring safety assessment. In addition, if any health messages are intended to be used also health claim regulations apply. This chapter reviews the regulatory settings and studies human milk oligosaccharides are required to fulfill to be able to enter markets in European Union or United States or elsewhere. Examples include Lacto-N-neotetraose and 2-fucosyllactose with safety assessment in European Union and United States.

Introduction

Human milk oligosaccharides (HMOs) are a group of sugars which are structurally diverse unconjugated glycans. They are found in human milk with a composition unique to each lactating mother [1]. They have not been used in any other foods previously, and, therefore, the supplementation of HMOs to our food requires both safety assessments and most likely assessment of potential health benefits, too [2–5].

While HMOs have been shown to have an impact on the development of infant gut microbiota, it is not well known if HMOs also already affect human milk microbiota composition or microbiota in oral, nasopharyngeal, gastrointestinal, and urinary tract areas [6, 7]. However, they do have a role in the early colonization of infant gut, and also a modifying and potentially protecting role specific to the mother and infant during pregnancy and breastfeeding [8]. HMOs are currently regarded as new ingredients for infant formulas, other foods, and food supplements. Such consideration involves specific regulatory steps, which are in process in several countries and regions.

Issues pertaining to novel HMOs have increased rapidly due to the fast-paced research on the impact HMOs and the possibility of their larger-scale production. HMOs represent novel tools to modulate the gut microbiota and thus potentially provide health benefits for infants, children, and adults. Such food ingredients are in demand as the importance of the gut microbiota on health has been stressed. HMOs could be considered as prebiotics, and specific components targeted toward unique outcomes and functionalities can be expected to emerge.

Regulatory Framework

In the majority of countries, HMOs are characterized as novel foods in the food regulation, and, therefore, several food authorities require a mandatory safety assessment.

The regulations governing the introduction of novel foods vary by geographical region. In some cases, confusion can result in differentiating novel foods from functional foods, or, as in the European Union, the regulatory category of functional foods is formed by foods with European Commission-approved health claims. The fundamental difference between these two categories of foods is that novel foods must be evaluated based on their safety, whereas foods with health claims need to be evaluated for any desired nutritional, functional, or disease risk reduction claims. Figure 1 demonstrates that the terms are distinct, but sometimes foods and food ingredients fall in both categories, which then necessitate evaluation for both safety and efficacy. The 2-category evaluation in Europe appears most likely for HMOs.

The views and challenges of current legislative framework in the USA, Europe, and some other countries are summarized regarding the assessment of HMOs and their novel food status from the regulatory and scientific viewpoint. Additionally, the possibility of future health claims is discussed.

HMOs are intrinsic components to manipulate the gut microbiota by providing an energy source for beneficial intestinal microbiota and potentially acting as decoy molecules to inactivate potential and opportunistic pathogens in the

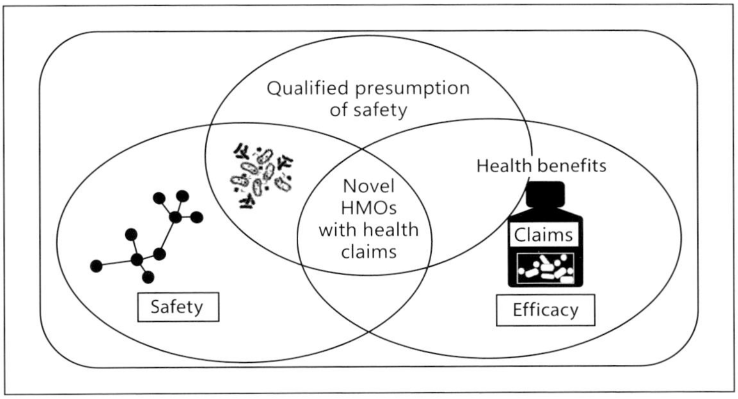

Fig. 1. European regulatory areas on novel foods and foods with health claims related to potential HMO-containing foods.

mucosal surfaces for improving the health of the host. Health-promoting outcomes are in demand as the importance of the gut microbiota in human health has been revealed. The regulations governing the introduction of HMOs vary by geographical region. Novel foods and foods with health claims fall under specific regulations in several countries. The main requirements of the regulations in the EU and USA are similar, but the approval processes differ. There are a number of areas that need to be addressed in any safety assessment of novel food ingredients (NFI).

European Union

Worldwide, the regulations governing novel foods, functional foods, and traditional foods vary. In the EU, the introduction of novel foods that have not been used in the EU prior to May 15, 1997, is currently governed by the Novel Food Regulation (EC) 285/97 [5]. This Regulation clearly defines the risk assessment steps required for any authorization of a novel food prior to the introduction into the EU market. It also defines the concept "substantial equivalence" to commonly used foods, in which case a simplified notification procedure applies. It also defines the role of EU Member States in the approval process. One Member State is responsible for the initial safety assessment of the novel food. Other Member States often challenge the initial assessment, or they ask additional questions related to the safety of novel foods. In these cases, concerns are usually discussed and answered by the European Food Safety Authority (EFSA) committee evaluations. Finally, the authorization decision is made either by the

Member State in lead or the European Commission with all Member States involved. In both cases, the authorization is valid allover the EU.

The Novel Food Regulation from 1997 has been under revision and the new regulation steps into force fully from January 2018 onwards. The most relevant change is the transfer to a fully centralized system in the EU. Dossiers are submitted to the European Commission, the EFSA is responsible for the safety assessment, and all authorizations are general, i.e. applicable for everybody without further notification. Changes in the update of the regulation cover also traditional foods from third-world countries. Currently, there is a transition period of 2 years during which the earlier mechanisms are still operable.

Current Regulation until 2018

Based on the current regulation, competent authorities of the member states and the European Commission assess if a food or food ingredient has no history of safe use prior to 1997 in Europe and hence is to be identified as "novel." The regulation then requires an extensive safety assessment of the food or ingredient prior to acceptance to the EU market [4]. A list of authorized novel foods and NFIs is available in the public registry by the EC. The decisions are explained in an inventory specifying the uses and restrictions for each novel food or novel food component, process, or NFI (http://ec.europa.eu/food/safety/novel_food/authorisations/list_authorisations/index_en.htm). For bacteria added to foods, which could also be considered novel, there is an annually updated list of microbes intentionally added to foods (QPS, Qualified Presumption of Safety of Microorganisms in Food and Feed), and this list forms the basis of organisms at the species level which are considered safe for foods and feeds in the EU (EFSA 2016 update). Due to their impact on microbiota, human milk oligosaccharide safety assessment may partly be related to microbiota as well.

A novel prebiotic can potentially be a component of conventional foods, food supplements, or foods for particular nutritional uses. Foods incorporating novel ingredients comprise also those designed for specific dietary requirements and may include infant and follow-on formulas, processed cereal-based food, food for special medical purposes, and total diet replacement for weight control.

Current Human Milk Oligosaccharides with Regulatory Decision in the European Union

Until now, 2 HMOs have gone through the novel food safety assessment in Europe with a positive assessment outcome and approval by the European Commission.

2′-O-Fucosyllactose (2′-FL) is a synthetic trisaccharide consisting of L-fucose, D-galactose, and D-glucose, which is produced by using L-fucose and

D-lactose as starting raw material. The NFI is intended by the applicant to be used in infant and follow-on formulae, foods for special medical purposes for infants and young children, and other foods for infants and young children. The NFI is also intended to be used in foods or food supplements for adults [3].

Lacto-N-neotetraose (LNnT) is a synthetic tetrasaccharide consisting of D-galactose, N-acetyl-D-glucosamine, D-galactose, and D-glucose, which is produced by using D-lactose as a starting raw material. The NFI is intended by the applicant to be used in infant and follow-on formulae, foods for special medical purposes for infants and young children, and other foods for infants and young children. The NFI is also intended to be used in foods or food supplements for adults [4].

A third safety assessment evaluation has been made by EFSA for the 2′-O-fucosyllactose in combination with lacto-N-neotetraose as a food supplement for children [5].

What Did the Member States Question in Case of Human Milk Oligosaccharides?

Several questions were raised by the EU member states following initial safety assessment. These included for example the following:

2′-O-Fucosyllactose [4]

- In the dossier, it is stated that the intake of 2′-FL in the form of food supplements would not be expected to influence the overall daily intake. However, one should consider the possibility for combined intake of 2′-FL from food supplements and other food uses specified in the dossier as a realistic scenario, which could more or less double the daily intake for high-level users.
- Considering that the NFI may also be consumed by more vulnerable individuals such as those with conditions that result in a "leaky gut," any further information could be provided on any possible consequences that may be associated with an increased level of NFI absorption.
- Intake of large quantities of indigestible carbohydrates may produce laxative effects. As there are no human studies on 2′-FL, apart from experience with infants who have been breastfed, nothing can be said about the quantities of 2′-FL which may produce laxative effects.
- The potential for genotoxicity was only assessed in 2 in vitro tests for mutagenicity. A test for potential clastogenic activity is lacking (in vitro micronucleus test or in vitro chromosome aberration test). The absence of genotoxicity for this 2′-FL preparation would only be demonstrated sufficiently upon obtaining a favorable outcome in such study.

Lacto-N-Neotetraose [5]

- Request confirmation that the solvents used are acceptable for food use.
- The estimated intake for distinct population groups, based on food consumption data from the UK, ranges from 26 to 329 mg/kg body weight per day for the 95th percentile. However, these intake estimates do not include the potential additional intake of LNnT from food supplements, as proposed in the application.
- The intake of large quantities of indigestible carbohydrates can have laxative effects. Since there are not yet any human studies on LNnT other than those with breastfed infants, no statement can be made on what levels of LNnT intake could potentially lead to laxative effects.

Nutrition and Health Claims

The EC regulation on nutrition and health claims 1924/2006 requires that such claims are based on scientific evidence and acceptability. EFSA has provided scientific and technical guidance for presenting applications for health claims on food [9]. Recently, an EFSA guidance document [10] or document on PARNUTS Directive 2009/39/EC or EU Regulation 609/2013 indicates that there are no escape routes to circumvent the Health Claims Regulation 1924/2006. Hendriksen and Verhagen [11] have developed a decision tree to discern PARNUTS foods from ordinary foods (with health claims). Following the publication of the Health Claims Regulation 1924/2006, the EFSA has evaluated around 3,000 health claims for scientific substantiation.

United States

In the United States, all foods and food ingredients are regulated under the Food Drug and Cosmetic Act (FDCA). In the USA, the safety of new and novel foods (including HMOs) is primarily the responsibility of the food manufacturer. The regulation states that:

> any substance that is intentionally added to food is a food additive that is subject to premarket review and approval by the Food and Drug Administration (FDA), unless the substance is generally recognized, among qualified experts, as having been adequately shown to be safe under the conditions of its intended use.

In the USA, HMOs intended for use in foods other than dietary supplements are regulated under the same regimen as all other food ingredients – that is, they may be introduced as food additives or as GRAS (Generally Recognized as Safe) substances, at the discretion of the manufacturer. There are two other conditions that pertain to GRAS substances. First, the information demonstrating safety must be generally available to the scientific community, usually regarded as requiring publication in the peer-reviewed scientific literature. Second, there must be general acceptance of the safety of the substances throughout the scientific community – there cannot be significant dispute regarding safety.

The FDA has no fundamental role in GRAS determinations except in an advisory capacity. The law that established GRAS (the 1958 Food Additive Amendment to the FDCA) specifically excluded GRAS substances from requiring FDA review and approval prior to entry into the food supply. The GRAS status of the intended use of a HMO is determined by a panel of qualified scientists who render the opinion that there is a "reasonable certainty of no harm" from the intended use, and further that they believe that other equally qualified scientists would reach the same conclusion. This process may be internal to the company and maintained as confidential to the company and disclosed only to customers under confidentiality.

In 1997, the law was amended to provide for a GRAS notification whereby companies could submit it to the FDA. The submission usually consists of an assessment of existing data by a group of recognized experts. Such safety assessment through scientific procedures requires the same quantity and quality of scientific evidence as is required to obtain approval of the substance as a food additive and ordinarily is based on published studies, which may be corroborated by unpublished studies and other data and information. This is a voluntary submission whereby the FDA reviews the information and the favorable FDA response is "FDA has no questions at this time."

HMOs have a long history of use in food for infants in human milk. However, the compositions vary, and HMOs are not available in other foods. For new and novel HMOs, the route to market as a dietary supplement is to have GRAS self-affirmed for use in food and then to use it in a dietary supplement in the same form. Such notifications have been provided for the 2′-O-fucosyllactose, 2′-fucosyllactose, and lacto-N-neotetraose:

2′-O-Fucosyllactose (Glycom A/S). Intended for use in term infant formula at a maximum level of 2,400 milligrams/Liter. Also intended for use in baked goods and baking mixes, beverages and beverages bases, coffee and tea, dairy product analogs, infant and toddler foods, grain products and pastas, milk (whole and skim), processed fruits and juices, processed vegetables and juices, and sugar substitutes at maximum levels ranging from 0.084 to 2.4 grams/serving [12].

2′-Fucosyllactose (Jennewein Biotechnologie, GmbH). For use as an ingredient in infant and toddler formula at a level of not more than 2 grams 2′-fucosyllactose per liter of formula [13].

Lacto-N-Neotetraose (Glycom A/S). Intended for use in term infant formula at a maximum level of 600 milligrams (mg)/Liter. Also intended for use in baked goods and baking mixes, beverages and beverage bases, coffee and tea, dairy product analogs, infant and toddler foods, grain products and pastas, milk (whole and skim), processed fruits and juices, processed vegetables and juices, and sugar substitutes at maximum levels ranging from 0.02 to 1.2 grams/serving [14].

Japan

In Japan, the assessment of novelty is based on both the source and the traditional use of foods or food ingredients in Japan. Details on novel HMOs are not available currently.

Australia

No applications of HMOs have been handled as of yet (August 2016).

Potential Areas for Health Claim Documentation

Several in vitro and even human studies have been conducted to foresee the potential of HMOs for health claims in Europe and the USA. An example of health claim substantiation is given for probiotics and prebiotics [15]. It is important to remember that the single HMOs and their combinations all form unique products for testing, and thus careful consideration and adjustment are necessary prior to conducting human intervention trials.

The areas of interest have included HMOs and necrotizing enterocolitis, different microbial challenges in the gut, traveller's diarrhea, and even long-term potentiation of learning capabilities in a rodent model [16–20].

Summary and Future Perspectives

What is known of HMOs in the regulatory area in the United States and the European Union:

- In the EU, HMOs are considered novel foods/NFIs with 2 oligosaccharides, and their combination passed through safety assessment.
- In the USA, 3 HMOs have been passed through according to the GRAS notification system.
- In the EU, the Novel Food Regulation is updated and will be fully operational in 2018; the approval system will be revised, and new guidance for applications has been set by EFSA.

Subject Index